Brit Long • Alex Koyfman

Editors

Handbook of Emergency Ophthalmology

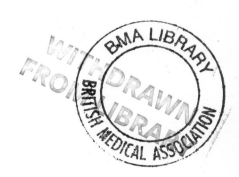
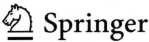 Springer

Editors
Brit Long
Department of Emergency
Medicine
San Antonio Military Medical
Center
Fort Sam Houston
TX
USA

Alex Koyfman
Department of Emergency
Medicine
The University of Texas
Southwestern Medical Center
Dallas
TX
USA

ISBN 978-3-319-78944-6   ISBN 978-3-319-78945-3   (eBook)
https://doi.org/10.1007/978-3-319-78945-3

Library of Congress Control Number: 2018945612

This Springer imprint is published by Springer Nature, under the registered company Springer International Publishing AG part of Springer Nature
The registered company address is: Gewerbestrasse 11, 6330 Cham, Switzerland

Preface

The sky is the daily bread for the eyes. — Ralph Waldo Emerson

I think that the greatest gift God ever gave man is not the gift of sight but the gift of vision. Sight is a function of eyes, but vision is a function of the heart. — Myles Munroe

Few are those who see with their own eyes and feel with their own hearts. — Albert Einstein

Emergency physicians are masters of evaluating and managing life-threatening diseases in the chaotic setting of the emergency department. We care for patients from different walks of life with many different symptoms and concerns. One of the most challenging organ systems emergency physicians manage is the ophthalmologic system. As the quotes describe above, the eyes are vital to normal function and daily life.

Many emergency physicians feel challenged with patients presenting with ophthalmologic symptoms, including eye pain, redness, swelling, or vision decrease/loss. The ophthalmologic examination contains various components with specialized equipment. Conditions may present no threat to the eyes, such as allergic conjunctivitis, or result in complete loss of vision such as retinal detachment or acute angle closure glaucoma. Many of these emergent conditions require immediate ophthalmologic specialist management.

This text, *Handbook of Emergency Ophthalmology,* presents a focused breakdown of the ophthalmologic history, examination, medications, conditions, and management, with the aim to provide emergency physicians, residents, medical students, nurses, and other healthcare workers vital information for the evaluation and management of the patient with an ophthalmologic condition.

We thank all of the authors involved in the construction of this book. We greatly appreciate the assistance of the staff at Springer. We also extend our gratitude to our families for their amazing support and patience during the writing and editing phases. We hope this book improves your clinical knowledge and practice, and thanks for reading!

San Antonio, TX, USA   Brit Long, MD
Dallas, TX, USA   Alex Koyfman, MD

Contents

Contributors

Paul Basel, MD Department of Emergency Medicine, San Antonio Uniformed Services Health Education Consortium, San Antonio, TX, USA

Ian Bodford, MD St. Francis Hospital, Memphis, TN, USA

Walter Green, MD Department of Emergency Medicine, University of Texas Southwestern Medical School, Dallas, TX, USA

Alex Koyfman, MD The University of Texas Southwestern Medical Center, Department of Emergency Medicine, Dallas, TX, USA

E. Liang Liu, MD Department of Emergency Medicine, UT Southwestern Medical Center, Dallas, TX, USA

Brit Long, MD San Antonio Military Medical Center, Department of Emergency Medicine, San Antonio, TX, USA

Brian Patrick Murray, DO Emergency Medicine, Brooke Army Medical Center, San Antonio, TX, USA

Patrick C. Ng, MD San Antonio Military Medical Center, Department of Emergency Medicine, San Antonio, TX, USA

Joshua J. Oliver, MD San Antonio Military Medical Center, Department of Emergency Medicine, San Antonio, TX, USA

Ashley Phipps, MD Department of Emergency Medicine, UT Southwestern Medical Center, Dallas, TX, USA

Daniel Reschke, MD Emergency Medicine, San Antonio Uniformed Services Health Education Consortium, San Antonio, TX, USA

Natalie Sciano, MD Emergency Department, University of Texas Southwestern Medical Center, Dallas, TX, USA

Matthew Streitz, MD Department of Emergency Medicine, San Antonio Uniformed Services Health Education Consortium, San Antonio, TX, USA

James L. Webb, MD San Antonio Uniformed Services Health Education Consortium, San Antonio, TX, USA

Dustin Williams, MD UT Southwestern Medical Center, Dallas, TX, USA

Chapter 1
Anatomy of the Eye

Patrick C. Ng and Joshua J. Oliver

The eye is a complex organ. Understanding the anatomy of the eye is helpful in understanding different pathologies, both medical and traumatic, that the emergency provider may be tasked with managing. This chapter will discuss the basic anatomy of the eye and its surrounding structures, focusing on the most pertinent structures for the emergency medicine differential diagnosis.

The External Structures

From external examination, there are several important structures to know (Fig. 1.1). Using a systematic approach, one should inspect the upper and lower eyelids, which provide protection and help maintain a tear film and protection for the eye [1].

Some important structures are revealed with the eye open (Fig. 1.2). The fold of the superior tarsal plate is best appreciated with the eye open and has implications with lacerations and other eye trauma. The sclera also known as the "white of

P. C. Ng, MD (✉) · J. J. Oliver, MD
San Antonio Military Medical Center, Department of Emergency Medicine, San Antonio, TX, USA

© Springer International Publishing AG, part of Springer Nature 2018
B. Long, A. Koyfman (eds.), *Handbook of Emergency Ophthalmology*, https://doi.org/10.1007/978-3-319-78945-3_1

Temporal Side   Nasal Side

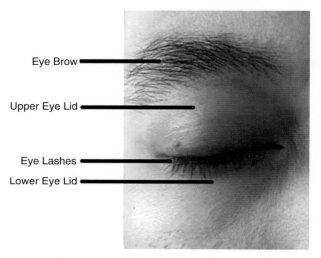

FIGURE 1.1 External eye closed

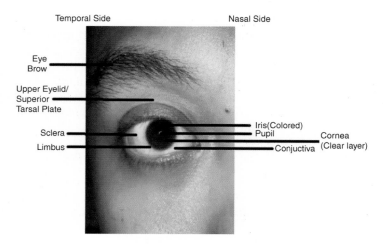

FIGURE 1.2 External eye open

the eye" is a protective layer of the outer eye made of fibrous tissue [2]. It can change color with certain disease processes including but not limited to hepatitis and/or liver failure. The cornea is a transparent layer of tissue that covers the pupil and iris (colored part of the eye) [3]. The limbus is where the cornea joints the sclera and can become injected with different disease processes. The pupil is an opening in the middle of the iris that is normally round. Elliptical or unequal pupil size can be consistent with trauma, different pathology, or prior surgeries [4].

There are several important structures located in the medial portion of the eye (Fig. 1.3). There are two pores located on the upper and lower medial lids called the puncta. They are small openings that allow tears to flow from the

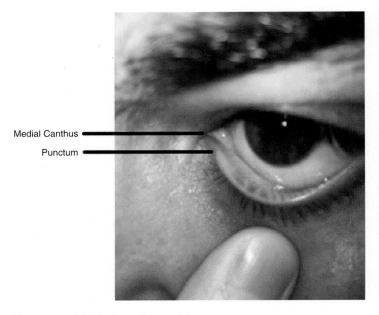

FIGURE 1.3 Medical canthus and lower punctum

lacrimal system to the anterior eye [5]. These structures can get clogged or damaged during trauma [6, 7]. It is important for the emergency provider to examine this structure in various clinical scenarios to ensure its patency. Lacerations involving the punctum require ophthalmologic consultation for repair as stenting of the canalicular system may be indicated (Fig. 1.4).

Anatomy of the lacrimal system

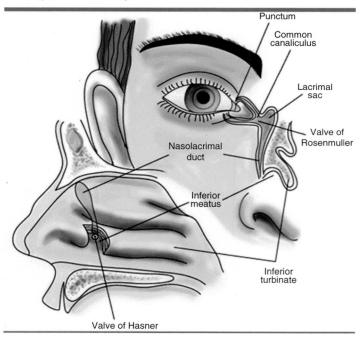

FIGURE 1.4 Canalicular system (Reproduced with permission from G Gardiner MF, Shah A. Approach to eye injuries in the emergency department. In: UpToDate, Post TW (Ed), UpToDate, Waltham, MA. (Accessed on 14 April 2016) Copyright © 2016 UpToDate, Inc. For more information, visit www.uptodate.com)

The Eyeball: Anterior Segment

The eyeball itself can be divided into an anterior and posterior segment (Fig. 1.5). The anterior segment contains the anterior chamber and posterior chamber, both of which contain aqueous humor. The anterior chamber is the area located between the cornea and iris. The posterior segment is behind the iris. Aqueous humor flows between the posterior chamber and the anterior chamber [8] (Fig. 1.6). When this drainage system becomes compromised, flow of aqueous humor can be disrupted leading to glaucoma [9].

The Eyeball: Posterior Segment and Layers of the Eye

The eyeball is composed of three layers, the sclera, the choroid, and the retina. The retina is composed of several layers of tissue, containing rods and cones. The retina recognizes light from the anterior portion of the eye, which then communicates with the CNS to form an image [10]. Various pathologies involving the retina can present with changes in vision, and it is important for the emergency medicine provider to promptly recognize these disease processes to minimize and prevent any permanent vision loss [11].

The retina can be directly visualized with a funduscopic exam. Important structures to recognize include the optic cup/disc, arteries and veins, as well as the macula. Evaluation of the optic cup/disc can be a sign of increased intraocular/intracranial pressure [12]. Examination of the arteries and veins are important in recognizing pathologies such as central retinal vein occlusion/central retinal artery occlusion in patients with acute vision changes [13]. The macula is a dark yellow/red oval structure on the retina. Within this structure, there is a dense concentration of photoreceptors and it is important in visual acuity. This structure is particularly important to recognize when suspecting pathology such as a retinal detachment which is when there is a tear in the retina

Horizontal section of the eyeball

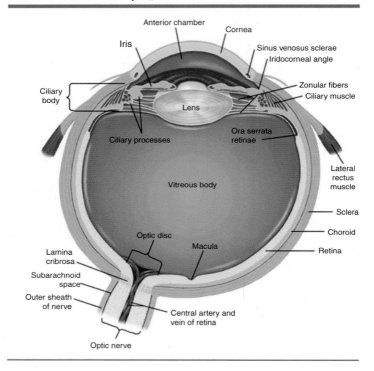

FIGURE 1.5 Cross section of eyeball. Representation of a horizontal section of the eyeball reveals its three coats: (1) external or fibrous coat (sclera and cornea); (2) middle or vascular coat (choroid, ciliary body, and iris); and (3) internal or retinal layer. The four refractive media are the cornea, the aqueous humor in the anterior chamber, the lens, and the vitreous body (Reproduced with permission from G Gardiner MF, Shah A. Approach to eye injuries in the emergency department. In: UpToDate, Post TW (Ed), UpToDate, Waltham, MA. (Accessed on 14 April 2016) Copyright © 2016 UpToDate, Inc. For more information, visit www.uptodate.com)

and fluid separates the retina from the posterior structures [14, 15]. The posterior segment of the eye contains a vitreous body which contains a gel-like substance called vitreous humor. In a normal eye, the vitreous body is adjacent to the

Glaucoma: Angle anatomy of the eye

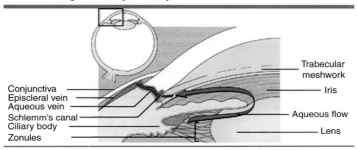

FIGURE 1.6 Flow of aqueous humor. The angle is the recess formed by the irido-corneal juncture. The scleral spur, trabecular meshwork, and Schwalbe's line lie within this angle. The trabecular meshwork is a fenestrated structure that transmits aqueous fluid to Schlemm's canal, from which it drains into the venous system. The normal flow of aqueous is demonstrated here (Reproduced with permission from Trobe JD. The Physician's Guide to Eye Care. Foundation of the American Academy of Ophthalmology, San Francisco, 2001. p. 158. Copyright © American Academy of Ophthalmology)

retina. When the vitreous body separates from the retina, it is called a posterior vitreous detachment (PVD), which can cause vision changes [16].

The Muscles of the Eye

There are six extraocular muscles that are involved in the movement of the eye (Fig. 1.7). The superior oblique muscle is involved in intorsion (rotation of the top of the eye toward the nose) and depression, while the inferior oblique is involved in extortion (rotation of the top of the eye away from the nose and elevation of the eye). The inferior rectus primarily moves the eye downward and the superior rectus primarily moves the eye upward. The lateral rectus is involved in abduction or movement of the eye away from the nose, while the medial rectus is involved with inward movement or adduction of the eye [16]. This group of muscles is innervated by cranial nerve (CN) III, IV, and VI

Extraocular muscles

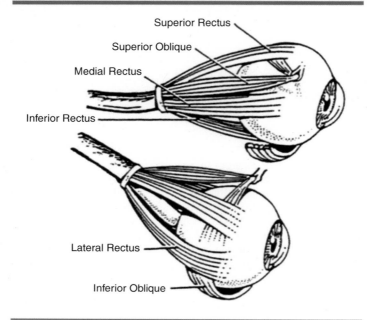

Superior Rectus

Superior Oblique

Medial Rectus

Inferior Rectus

Lateral Rectus

Inferior Oblique

FIGURE 1.7 Extraocular muscles of the eye. Each eye has six extra-ocular muscles, which are yoked in pairs (Reproduced with permission from: Lavin, PJM. Eye movement disorders and diplopia. In: Neurology in clinical practice: Principles of Diagnosis and Management, 2nd ed, Bradley, WG (Ed), Butterworth-Heinemann, Boston 1996. p. 185. Copyright © 1996 Elsevier)

TABLE 1.1
Extraocular
muscles and
innervations

Muscle	Innervation
Superior oblique	CN IV (trochlear)
Inferior oblique	CN III (oculomotor)
Superior rectus	CN III (oculomotor)
Inferior rectus	CN III (oculomotor)
Medial rectus	CN III (oculomotor)
Lateral rectus	CN VI (abducens)

(Table 1.1). Understanding this group of muscles and their innervations is essential as extraocular muscle dysfunction/palsy can be indicative of different disease processes such as, but not limited to, ischemia, giant cell arteritis, aneurysms, and malignancy [17].

Muscles Surrounding the Eye

The muscles surrounding the eye include the orbicularis oculi, frontalis, and levator palpebrae superioris. The levator palpebrae superioris is involved in the movement of the superior tarsal plate and, like some of the extraocular muscles, is innervated by CN III. A drooping eyelid can be suggestive of pathology involving CN III and this muscle [18–21].

Bony Structures of the Eye

There are seven bones that form the orbit, which is a bony structure that the eye ball sits in (Fig. 1.8). Posterior to the eyeball is the sphenoid bone. Lateral is the zygomatic bone. Inferior and lateral borders are composed of the maxillary, lacrimal, ethmoid, and palatine bones. Lastly, the frontal bone forms the superior portion of the orbit. These structures are important to know, particularly in the setting of facial trauma. Trauma to the orbit can result in "blowout" fractures which can present with entrapment of an extraocular muscle. Patients with this pathology can have limited range of motion of the eyeball depending on which muscle may be affected. This is important for the emergency physician to recognize and manage with expert consultation with a facial trauma surgeon [22–25].

Bones of the orbit

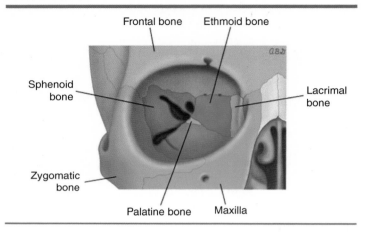

FIGURE 1.8 Bones of the orbit (Reproduced with permission from G Gardiner MF, Shah A. Approach to eye injuries in the emergency department. In: UpToDate, Post TW (Ed), UpToDate, Waltham, MA. (Accessed on 14 April 2016) Copyright © 2016 UpToDate, Inc. For more information, visit www.uptodate.com)

Conclusion

An understanding of eye anatomy is central to evaluation and management of ophthalmologic conditions. Ophthalmologic anatomy includes the external structures, anterior and posterior eyeball, ocular musculature within and outside the eye, and bony structures of the eye. A more detailed anatomy will be discussed in the context of different disease processes in other sections of this text.

References

1. Cunningham ET, Riorda-Eva P. Vaugh & Asbury's general ophthalmology. 18th ed. New York: McGraw Hill Medical; 2011.
2. Cassin B, Solomon S. Dictionary of eye terminology. Gainesville, FL: Triad; 1990.

3. Dua HS, Faraj LA, Said DG, Gray T, Lowe J. Human corneal anatomy redefined. Ophthalmology. 2013;120(9):1778–85.
4. Gamm DM, Albert DM. Pupil. https://www.britannica.com/science/pupil-eye. Last Accessed 23 July 2016.
5. Hurwitz JJ, Corin SM, Tucker SM. Punctal and vertical canaliculus lacerations. Ophthalmic Surg. 1989;20(7):514–6.
6. Seiff SR, Shorr N. Nasolacrimal drainage system obstruction after orbital decompression. Am J Ophthalmol. 1988;106(2):204–9.
7. Ophthobook.com. http://www.ophthobook.com/chapters/anatomy. Last Accessed 24 July 2016.
8. Braakman ST, Moore JE, Ethier CR, Overby DR. Transport across Schlemm's canal endothelium and the blood-aqueous barrier. Exp Eye Res. 2016;146:17–21.
9. Chowdhury UR, Hann CR, Stamer WD, Fautsch MP. Aqueous humor outflow: dynamics and disease. Invest Ophthalmol Vis Sci. 2015;56(5):2993–3003.
10. Heavner W, Pevny L. Eye development and retinogenesis. Cold Spring Harb Perspect Biol. 2012;4(12):a008391.
11. Alangh M, Chaudhary V, McLaughlin C, Chan B, Mullen SJ, Barbosa J. Ophthalmic referrals from emergency wards—a study of cases referred for urgent eye care (the R.E.S.C.U.E study). Can J Ophthalmol. 2016;51(3):174–9.
12. Park HY, Kim SE, Park CK. Optic disc change during childhood myopic shift: comparison between eyes with an enlarged cup-to-disc ratio and childhood glaucoma compared to normal myopic eyes. PLoS One. 2015;10(7):e0131781.
13. Kurtz WS, Glueck CJ, Hutchins RK, Sisk RA, Wang P. Retinal artery and vein thrombotic occlusion during pregnancy: markers for familial thrombophilia and adverse pregnancy. Clin Ophthalmol. 2016;10:935–8.
14. Yanoff M, Sassani JW. Ocular pathology. Maryland Heights, MI: Mosby; 2009.
15. Joe SG, Kim YJ, Chae JB, Yang SJ, Lee JY, Kim JG, et al. Structural recovery of the detached macula after retinal detachment repair as assessed by optical coherence tomography. Korean J Ophthalmol. 2013;27(3):178–85.
16. Montgomery TM. Anatomy, physiology and pathology of the human eye. http://www.tedmontgomery.com/the_eye/indexeom.html. Last Accessed 29 July 2016.
17. King NH, Stavem GP. Isolated ocular motor nerve palsies. Semin Neurol. 2015;35:539–48.

18. Santos T, Morais H, Oliveira G, Barros P. Isolated oculomotor nerve palsy, a rare manifestation of internal carotid artery dissection. BMJ Case Rep. 2014;16:2014.
19. Bagheri A, Borhani M, Salehirad S, Yazdani S, Tavakoli M. Blepharoptosis associated with third cranial nerve palsy. Ophthal Plast Reconstr Surg. 2015;31(5):357–60.
20. Tsuda H, Fujita T, Maruyama K, Ishihara M. Claude's syndrome without ptosis caused by a midbrain infaction. Intern Med. 2015;54(14):1799–801.
21. Aliswaina N, Elkhamary SM, Shammari MA, Khan AO. Ophthalmic features of outpatient children diagnosed with intracranial space-occupying lesions by ophthalmologists. Middle East Afr J Ophthalmol. 2015;22(3):327–30.
22. Fujino T, Makino K. Entrapment mechanism and ocular injury in orbital blowout fracture. Plast Reconstr Surg. 1980;65(5):571–6.
23. Smith B, Regan WF. Blow-out fracture of the orbit; mechanism and correction of internal orbital fracture. Am J Ophthalmol. 1957;44(6):733–9.
24. Converse JM, Smith B. Enophthalmos and diplopia in fractures of the orbital floor. Br J Plast Surg. 1957;9:265–74.
25. Choi M, Roberto LF. Medial orbital wall fractures and the transcaruncular approach. J Craniofac Surg. 2012;23:696–701.

Chapter 2
Evaluating Eye Complaints

Brit Long and Alex Koyfman

Patients with ophthalmologic complaints can present with a variety of signs and symptoms including the red eye, pain, trauma, and vision loss. The ophthalmologic history and physical examination can provide the keys to diagnosis. This chapter will evaluate the important historical and physical examination maneuvers required in the ophthalmologic evaluation.

History

A detailed history is vital in the ophthalmologic evaluation. Several aspects of the history are important. The history and evaluation should first categorize the patient complaint including vision loss, eye pain, trauma, or change in the appearance of the eye. Eye pain or discomfort should include the type of pain (aching, throbbing, sharp, stabbing, etc.) or a foreign body sensation. Visual fields defects should be evalu-

B. Long, MD (✉)
San Antonio Military Medical Center, Department of Emergency Medicine, San Antonio, TX, USA

A. Koyfman, MD
The University of Texas Southwestern Medical Center, Department of Emergency Medicine, Dallas, TX, USA

© Springer International Publishing AG, part of Springer Nature 2018
B. Long, A. Koyfman (eds.), *Handbook of Emergency Ophthalmology*, https://doi.org/10.1007/978-3-319-78945-3_2

ated. Flashing lights or a curtain descending suggests retinal detachment. Sudden loss of vision suggests central retinal artery occlusion. Eye pain following trauma may be due to foreign body.

Other important aspects include the mechanism of injury or suspected etiology per the patient, time of symptom onset, and other coexisting complaints. Mechanism of injury is important, as is the time of symptom onset [1–3]. Patients should also be questioned about similar prior symptoms.

The patient's past medical history is important and can focus the examination and differential diagnosis. Previous ophthalmologic surgeries, corrective vision lens or glasses, and use of ophthalmologic medications should be questioned. Cardiac risk factors such as hypertension, diabetes mellitus, and hyperlipidemia are associated with certain ophthalmologic conditions. A history of other exposures or toxic ingestions should be obtained.

The following key questions must be asked:

1. What is the chief complaint(s): pain, visual disturbance, photophobia, discharge, or color change?
2. Did an object get in the eye, and is there any associated trauma?
3. Was there any chemical exposure?
4. Is there any previous eye history, including vision correction and prior ocular surgery?
5. Are corrective/contact lenses used?
6. Are infectious symptoms present?
7. Are there systemic signs or symptoms?

Physical Examination

After the focused history, a complete physical exam can provide a great deal of vital information. Many emergency physicians are uncomfortable completing ophthalmologic exams, but this is an essential aspect of the care we provide. The following should be assessed in the patient with visual loss [1–3].

Visual Acuity

This aspect of the physical examination is one of the most important, as visual acuity is considered the vital sign of the eye. This should be conducted before shining a bright light into the eye, which may affect visual acuity. Only in the setting of chemical burn to the eye should visual acuity testing be delayed for irrigation.

The Snellen eye chart is the most efficacious means of evaluating visual acuity. The patient should stand 20 feet from the chart. Visual acuity is measured by the smallest line a patient can read with one half correct. The visual acuity of each eye should be tested and documented separately and then together. If the patient requires correction at baseline, the patient's contact lenses or glasses should be used when testing. Otherwise a pinhole occlude should be used. If this is not available, a perforated note card or metal eye shield may be used. Visual acuity for near vision can be evaluated with a Rosenbaum chart.

If visual acuity is less than 20/200, finger counting or perception of movement should be tested. If this fails, light perception should be evaluated. Patients who are illiterate can be tested using the letter E and what direction the letter points. Children can be tested with an Allen chart, which contains pictures.

General Appearance

A gross inspection of the eyebrows, eyelids, and lacrimal apparatus should be conducted. The periorbital skin and eyelids could be closely evaluated for signs of trauma, laceration, irritation, proptosis, deformity, or erythema. The orbits should be palpated to evaluate for crepitus or deformities. The upper eyelid should then be everted to evaluate for foreign bodies using a cotton applicator, though this only visualizes the lower half of the upper eyelid. The inner part of upper lid will require an eyelid retractor to tent the upper lid. A paperclip can also be used in place of an eyelid retractor.

Visual Fields

Full vision contains four different quadrants, which should be evaluated. The examiner should have the patient close one eye and look at the examiner's nose, while the examiner closes the opposite eye. Either testing of movement or the number of fingers held in the peripheral vision field can be evaluated. Normal visual fields are observed when the patient sees the movement or number at the same time as the examiner.

Pupils

The size, shape, and reaction to light of each pupil should be assessed. Any irregularity in shape can be due to trauma or surgery, and the patient should be asked about prior knowledge of pupil irregularity. A tear drop pupil could be due to rupture of the globe or iris.

A pupil that does not respond to light, or an afferent pupillary defect, is a sign of optic nerve pathology. This defect is known as a Marcus Gunn pupil. Also, any pathology that prevents light from reaching the CNS can also cause an afferent pupillary defect. A swinging flashlight test will cause constriction of the ipsilateral pupil and consensual constriction of the opposite pupil. When the light is shined in the opposite, affected pupil, the affected pupil will dilate in the presence of an afferent pupillary defect.

Anisocoria, or unequal pupils, can range from physiologic to pathologic. Physiologic anisocoria is most common, with a difference of less than 1 mm in pupils. One dilated pupil can be due to uncal herniation, use of a topical cycloplegic agent, or pathology of the iris sphincter.

Extraocular Movements

Six cardinal positions of gaze exist, and six extraocular muscles attached to each eye control eye movements. Cranial nerves III, IV, and VI innervate these muscles. Cranial nerve III controls all extraocular muscles except the superior oblique muscle (cranial nerve IV) and the lateral rectus muscle (cranial nerve VI). Movement of the eyes can be impaired through several mechanisms including innervation, trauma, and restriction. Alignment should be evaluated first with the patient looking straight ahead (known as primary gaze), followed by eye movements in all fields.

Diplopia may be a sign of extraocular muscle pathology, which is worse when the patient looks in the direction of the deficient or affected muscle. If diplopia is present when one eye is covered, this is due to corneal pathology, lens disease, or malingering. If diplopia improves with covering one eye, this is suggestive of extraocular muscle pathology. Unfortunately a Wood's lamp may miss microscopic or punctate abrasions. Thus, a slit lamp is most efficacious and sensitive.

Anterior Chamber and Slit Lamp

The anterior chamber consists of the conjunctiva, sclera, cornea, iris, and ciliary body. The slit lamp is a binocular microscope that magnifies ocular structures. To use a slit lamp appropriately, the patient and examiner must be seated at the same level, and the slit lamp height must be at a level where the patient may lean forward and rest comfortably with the forehead against the upper bar and the chin on the bottom chin rest. The patient's lateral canthus should be even with the black line of the vertical bar.

The slit lamp's oculars and light source are straight ahead, and focus is adjusted by anterior/posterior movement of the light source using a joystick. Rotating the joystick controls vertical movement of the light source. The vertical light beam should be adjusted to the height of the cornea with a width of 1 mm. Magnification should be set at 1X to begin, with the light source 45° on the temporal side of the eye being assessed.

First examine the lids and conjunctivae for any signs of trauma, swelling, or inflammation. Scan across the upper and lower lids. The cornea is examined with the light source at 45° to the patient. The epithelium of the cornea should be examined for any signs of ulceration, abrasion, or trauma.

The depth of the anterior chamber can be examined by adjusting the angle of the light source. If the iris is bowed forward, a shadow appears on the nasal or medial iris. Evaluation for cell and flare should be conducted by shortening the slit beam to 1 mm and placing the magnification on high setting. The light beam should be focused on the pupillary margin, and the joystick can then be used to focus on the cornea. Keratic precipitates will appear as white spots on the corneal epithelium undersurface. The focus should then be moved inward the pupillary aperture as a black background. The focus will be placed in the center of the aqueous humor with this maneuver, which may demonstrate WBCs and RBCs slowly drifting. Flare appears like "headlights in a fog" and is caused by increased aqueous protein in the anterior chamber, often seen in inflammatory conditions. Iritis can result in WBC layers in the anterior chamber known as hypopyon, and RBC layers in the anterior chamber are known as hyphema. The iris should be evaluated for irregularity and dysfunction with the light beam as well.

There are several pitfalls that may occur with use of the slit lamp. If no light is present, ensure the machine is on. Some slit lamps require three switches in the "on" position. If focus is poor, try moving the joystick forward and back first, followed by adjustment of the eye pieces. Ensure the eye pieces have proper width for the examiner and proper focus. Also ensure the patient's forehead is resting against the upper plastic bar. If the light is difficult to aim, ensure the patient's eyes are level with the red line on the slit lamp.

Fluorescein

This is normally a component of the slit lamp examination, though it can also be completed with a woods lamp. Fluorescein is instilled into the eye, which will bind to damage epithelium on the cornea. Remove any contact lens before instilling fluorescein. Instilling fluorescein should be completed by applying eye irrigation solution or topic anesthetic drops to the strip, followed by lightly dabbing the end of the strip to the inferior conjunctival fornix. The patient should then blink several times to distribute the stain. The cornea can then be examined for streaming of fluorescein tinged aqueous humor, which is a positive Seidel test. Under a Wood's lamp or cobalt blue filter on the slit lamp, a corneal abrasion will fluoresce green.

Posterior Chamber

This aspect of the ophthalmologic examination can be difficult. Fundoscopy is the classic examination. When using fundoscopy, the patient should sit upright and look straight ahead. Dilatation with 1% tropicamide or 2.5% phenylephrine will assist viewing the disk, macula, and retinal vessels. Indirect ophthalmoscopy can be completed but is often difficult to obtain adequate images of the necessary structures. Direct ophthalmoscopy is most efficacious with a Welch Allyn Panoptic™ direct ophthalmoscope.

A Welch Allyn Panoptic™ direct ophthalmoscope allows greater view of the fundus and a better view of the fundus with an undilated pupil than a standard direct ophthalmoscope. This tool requires several key steps. (1) First have the patient sit upright and remove any glasses (examiner and/or patient). With the scope in the off position, focus on an object 10 feet away. (2) Then set the aperture dial to small, and turn on the scope to maximal brightness. (3) Have the patient sit still and continue to look straight ahead. Warn the patient the eyecup will touch the patient. (4) The examiner should be place his or her on the patient's forehead with the scope positioned 6 inches away at a 20° angle to the temporal side. (5) The red light reflex should be located, and then the scope is moved toward the patient with the light reflex in view. (6) Maximum view will be obtained with the eyecup is compressed by half.

When using a direct-held ophthalmoscope, the size and shape of the optic disk, cut-to-disk ratio, and size ratio of the arteries to veins should be evaluated. The normal size ratio of artery to vein is 2:3. The texture and color of the retina, size and color of the macula, and lens appearance should be assessed. Inability to evaluate these structures is likely due to lens opacities or lesions in the vitreous. Papilledema refers to bilateral edema of the optic nerve head, due to increased intracranial pressure. This causes blurring of the disk margins, diminished or absent optic cup, and elevation of the nerve head.

Intraocular Pressure (IOP)

The eye constantly balances production and outflow of aqueous fluid. Intraocular pressure can increase when intraocular fluid production is greater than outflow. Pressure may decrease when production is reduced or with globe rupture. In the setting of globe rupture, intraocular pressure should not be measured. However, in all causes of vision loss, eye pain, or trauma with low suspicion of rupture, obtaining IOP measurements is warranted.

Normal IOP is 10–20 mm Hg. Palpation of the globe with the examiner's fingers can give an estimation of IOP, but for adequate measurement, a device that measures IOP is needed. Several devices include the Schiötz tonometer, Tono-Pen® XL (Reichert, Inc., Depew, NY), Goldmann® applanation tonometer, and pneumatonometer. These devices have overtaken the Schiötz tonometer due to ease of use and accuracy. Before using such a device, anesthetize the eye with a topic anesthetic. To measure pressure, keep the lids open with the examiner's fingers while the patient looks straight ahead. Do not place pressure on the globe with the fingers while holding the lids, as this can cause a falsely high reading.

The Tono-Pen® XL uses a disposable cover and is touched to the cornea four to eight times, followed by an average IOP. A Goldmann® applanation tonometer requires training before use and is used by optometrists and ophthalmologists.

In order to use the Tono-Pen® XL, first anesthetize the patient's cornea and calibrate the machine. Place the patient in a seated or supine position, and have him or her focus on a distant object. Touch the Tono-Pen® XL lightly and briefly to the cornea several times. A successful measurement will result in a high-pitched chirp. Only valid readings will result in this chirp, and an average will then be displayed. Ensure both eyes are evaluated using the Tono-Pen® XL to compare intraocular pressure.

Ocular Ultrasound (US)

Ocular US is discussed in detail in Chapter 14. This imaging modality is ideal for evaluating several eye emergencies. In many settings such as periorbital edema, corneal abrasion, and hyphema, the posterior chamber may be difficult to evaluate. Ocular US can be used in the evaluation of vision loss/decreased vision, ocular pain, trauma, head injury, assessment for elevated intracranial pressure, and suspected intraocular foreign body.

The technique involves using a 7.5–10 mHz linear array transducer under ocular settings. The patient should be supine of partially upright with the eyes closed. Water-soluble US gel should be generously applied to the patient's closed eyelid. The eye is then scanned in sagittal and transverse planes, while the patient looks straight ahead. Both eyes should be evaluated in neutral position and during movement of the eye under the closed eyelid.

A normal eye offers an optimal acoustic window, and the normal eye will be circular and hypoechoic. Pathologies such as lens dislocation, retrobulbar hematoma, foreign body, globe rupture, retinal detachment, vitreous hemorrhage, and elevated intracranial pressure may be discovered on US.

References

1. Nash EA, Margo CE. Patterns of emergency department visits for disorders of the eye and ocular adnexa. Arch Ophthalmol. 1998;116(9):1222–6.
2. Walker RA, Adhikaris. Eye emergencies. Tintinalli's emergency medicine: a comprehensive study guide. 8th ed. Pennsylvania: McGraw-Hill Education; 2016. Chap. 241.
3. Guluma K, Lee JE. Ophthalmology. Rosen's Emergency Meidcine: Concepts and Clinical Practice; 2016. Chap. 61, p. 790-819.e3.

Chapter 3
Ophthalmologic Medications

Brit Long

Emergency physicians provide a large amount of the ophthalmologic care in the United States, mostly for conditions other than trauma [1]. While emergency medicine physicians may possess comfort with ophthalmologic conditions, an array of medications and indications for medications in these complaints can result in discomfort with ophthalmologic medications. This chapter examines the different classes of emergent ophthalmological medications, including dosing and indications.

Anesthetics

Two types of anesthetics exist for use in ophthalmologic conditions: esters and amides. The most common esters are proparacaine (0.5%) and tetracaine (0.5%). Tetracaine lasts approximately 30 min once applied, in comparison to proparacaine which lasts 15 min and is slightly more irritating and slower in onset.
Color cap: White.

B. Long, MD
San Antonio Military Medical Center, Department
of Emergency Medicine, San Antonio, TX, USA

© Springer International Publishing AG, part of Springer
Nature 2018
B. Long, A. Koyfman (eds.), *Handbook of Emergency
Ophthalmology*, https://doi.org/10.1007/978-3-319-78945-3_3

Mechanism of action: Anesthetics function as sodium channel blockers, which decreases depolarization and action potential propagation.

Indications: Used for topical anesthesia, assisting with examination and procedures. These medications can be used to help differentiate corneal causes of symptoms versus other causes. Use in an outpatient setting is controversial for pain control; however, diluting the solution is feasible and likely will not cause delayed healing or toxicity [1–3].

Dosing: One to two drops in the ED.

Considerations: Recent literature supports increased patient satisfaction with local anesthetics within a 24 h period and no evidence of difference in corneal healing. Literature and FOAM resources support the use of diluting the 0.5% concentration into 0.05%. This can be done using a 10 cc flush, ejecting 1 cc of the saline, and replacing this with 1 cc of the anesthetic [4, 5].

Mydriatics and Cycloplegics

Mydriatics and cycloplegics function to dilate the eye. Mydriatic medications accomplish this by paralyzing the iris sphincter, which causes dilation without affecting accommodation. On the other hand, cycloplegics paralyze both the iris sphincter and the ciliary muscles, causing dilation and affecting accommodation. Phenylephrine (2.5%) is a common dilating agent with onset 15 min, lasting for 3–4 h. Cycloplegics are often used for conditions causing inflammation of the eye. Several cycloplegics include:

- Cyclopentolate has an onset of 30–60 min with duration of approximately 24 h.
- Tropicamide has an onset of 15–20 min with duration of approximately 6 h.
- Homatropine and atropine have a duration of days to weeks and probably have little role in the ED due to this length of action.

Color cap: Red.

Mechanism of action: Mydriatics are sympathomimetic agents that paralyze the iris sphincter. Cycloplegics are parasympatholytic agents that paralyze the iris sphincter and the ciliary muscles.

Indications: These medications are helpful for evaluating painless monocular vision complaints such as vision loss. They can be used to treat ciliary spasm, decreasing ocular pain, in iritis and deep corneal ulcers.

Dosing: One drop in the ED. These medications are usually required once per day if prescribed for home use.

Considerations: These medications are contraindicated in patients with suspicion for increased intraocular pressure, especially in acute angle closure glaucoma, as well as in the presence of shallow anterior chamber or concern for ruptured globe. Interestingly, blue-eyed individuals are more sensitive than brown-eyed individuals to mydriatics and cycloplegics.

Miotics (Cholinergic)

In emergency medicine, the most common use for miotic agents is acute angle closure glaucoma. The most common miotic is pilocarpine (2%), which facilitates drainage of the aqueous humor.

Color cap: Dark green.

Mechanism of action: Miotics cause pupillary constriction, pulling the iris back from an anterior position.

Indications: This class of medication is used in acute angle closure glaucoma.

Dosing: Two drops three to four times per day.

Considerations: In the ED, this medication will be used in acute angle closure glaucoma but is only efficacious once the intraocular pressure is less than 40 mm Hg. They should only be applied after initial measures are completed, and both eyes should be medicated with pilocarpine in the setting of acute angle closure glaucoma. In the setting of cataract surgery, it may be better to dilate the eye and avoid this agent.

Antimicrobials

Topical antibiotics are often overprescribed. However, they are indicated for a number of ophthalmic diagnoses including bacterial conjunctivitis, corneal ulcers, and blepharitis. Antibiotics are administered as either solutions or ointments. Drops are rapidly absorbed and require frequent instillation. Ointments have longer duration and require less frequent administration. However, they cause blurred vision when applied.

Color cap: Tan.

Mechanism of action: A variety of mechanisms exist for these medications. These are shown in Table 3.1.

Indications: As discussed previously, indications include bacterial conjunctivitis, corneal ulcers, and blepharitis.

Dosing: Usually dependent on specific agent, with one to two drops one to four times per day.

Considerations: Please see Table 3.1.

Topical antivirals (idoxuridine, trifluridine, and ganciclovir) are used for treatment of viral infection such as herpes simplex keratitis but should not be given without consultation with an ophthalmologist. Dosing includes one drop every hour for idoxuridine, one drop every 2 h for trifluridine, and one drop five times per day for ganciclovir (used to treat cytomegalovirus).

Antibiotic-steroid combination medications exist, but these should only be used in conjunction with ophthalmology.

Steroids

Topic steroids (prednisolone acetate, fluorometholone, and dexamethasone) are indicated only in specific circumstances. This class is contraindicated in the setting of ocular

TABLE 3.1 Specific antibiotic medications [6]

Class	Medication	Specifics
Macrolide	Erythromycin 0.5%	– Exists as ointment only, which is soothing – Covers gram-positive agents – Covers chlamydia trachomatis – Safe for newborns/infants – Not for contact lens users
Fluoroquinolone	Levofloxacin 1.5% Ciprofloxacin 0.3% Ofloxacin 0.3% Fourth-generation quinolones (moxifloxacin, gatifloxacin, besifloxacin)	– High resistance for early-generation medications, but improved with fourth generation – Expensive – Can be used in monotherapy for contact lens wearers and ulcers – Fourth-generation medications are expensive and have great gram-negative and *Pseudomonas* coverage – Fourth-generation medications do not have good streptococcal coverage

(continued)

TABLE 3.1 (continued)

Class	Medication	Specifics
Aminoglycoside	Tobramycin 0.3% Gentamicin 0.3%	– Gram-negative and streptococcal coverage – Useful for contact lens wearers
Other options	Bacitracin Polymyxin B/ trimethoprim Sulfacetamide	– Good gram-positive coverage, useful for blepharitis – Broad coverage – Useful in pediatric patients – Inhibits production of folic acid, useful for blepharitis

infection such as herpes simplex keratoconjunctivitis or bacterial infection. Use of this class warrants ophthalmologist consultation.

Color cap: Pink.

Mechanism of action: Decrease inflammation by inhibiting edema, leukocyte migration, fibrin deposition, and collagen deposition and scar formation.

Indications: These medications may be indicated in treatment of corneal injury from burns (chemical, thermal, radiation), allergic conjunctivitis, herpes zoster keratitis, punctate keratitis, iritis, and selected infective conjunctivitis.

Dosing: One to two drops twice daily.

Considerations: This class should only be used with ophthalmologic consultation. Topical corticosteroids can lead to cataracts, corneal thinning, glaucoma, and infection.

Adrenergic Agents

Topical adrenergic agents include beta-antagonists (timolol, betaxolol) and alpha-2-agonists (apraclonidine, brimonidine).

Beta Blockers

Color cap: Yellow.

Mechanism of action: These medications reduce intraocular pressure through decreasing aqueous humor secretion by the ciliary body.

Indications: This class is only used in the setting of acute angle closure glaucoma.

Dosing: One drop two to three times per day (once in the ED).

Considerations: The provider must be wary of cardiopulmonary effects including hypotension, syncope, heart block, and worsening of asthma. Of note, combination beta-blockers may have a dark blue cap.

Alpha Agonists

Color cap: Purple.

Mechanism of action: Similar to topical beta-blockers, these medications decrease aqueous humor production, decreasing intraocular pressure.

Indications: Acute angle closure glaucoma.

Dosing: One drop three times per day (once in the ED).

Combigan Ophthalmic Solution® is a combination and alpha-2 agonist and beta-blocker used for glaucoma, with one drop provided every 12 h.

Carbonic Anhydrase Inhibitors

Medications in this class include dorzolamide and brinzolamide (Trusopt and Azopt). They repress carbonic anhydrase, reducing pressure in the eye through reduction in aqueous humor production.

Color cap: Orange.

Mechanism of action: These medications reduce intraocular pressure through decreasing aqueous humor secretion by the ciliary body.

Indications: This class is only used in the setting of acute angle closure glaucoma.

Dosing: One drop three times per day.

Considerations: This class should not be used in patients with sickle disease or trait, which may lead to acute angle closure glaucoma.

Prostaglandin Analogues

This class consists of travoprost, latanoprost, bimatoprost, and tafluprost. These medications reduce intraocular pressure by increasing outflow of aqueous humor.

Color cap: Turquoise.

Mechanism of action: These medications reduce intraocular pressure through increasing outflow of aqueous humor.

Indications: This class is used for acute angle closure glaucoma.

Dosing: One drop dosed one to four times per day, specific to the agent used.

Considerations: The provider must be wary of cardiopulmonary effects including hypotension, syncope, heart block, and worsening of asthma.

Antihistamine/Decongestant

This medication class is useful for conjunctival congestion and pruritus. Medications include naphazoline and pheniramine (Naphcon-A® and Visine A®).

Color cap: Olive green [8, 9].

Mechanism of action: This class works as histamine receptor antagonists.

Indications: Medications are used for conjunctival congestion or pruritus.

Dosing: One drop two times per day.

Considerations: This class should not be used for over 72 h. They should be avoided in narrow angle glaucoma, hypertension, and contact lens use.

Nonsteroidal Anti-inflammatory Drugs

These medications provide another option for pain and inflammation control for ophthalmologic complaints. Medications include ketorolac, bromfenac, nepafenac, and diclofenac sodium.

Color cap: Gray [8, 9].

Mechanism of action: These agents reversibly inhibit cyclooxygenase-1 and cyclooxygenase-2 (COX-1 and COX-2 enzymes), which decrease formation of prostaglandin. They also decrease cytokine levels and immune cellular activation.

Indications: This class can be used in allergic conjunctivitis, corneal abrasions, and UV keratitis.

Dosing: Dependent on the specific agent. Ketorolac and diclofenac are given one drop three to four times per day, while bromfenac is given one drop per day.

Considerations: These agents may enhance topical glucocorticoid effects.

Mast Cell Stabilizers

These agents are primarily used in the setting of allergic conjunctivitis. Medications include nedocromil sodium (Alocril Ophthalmic Solution®), pemirolast potassium (Alamast Ophthalmic Solution®), lodoxamide tromethamine (Alomide Ophthalmic Solution®), and cromolyn sodium (Cromolyn Sodium Ophthalmic Solution®). These medications are not useful for acute symptoms, as full efficacy is not reached until at least 5 days of use [7].

Mechanism of action: This medication class functions to stabilize mast cell membranes, preventing the release of histamine and leukotrienes.

Indications: These are used for allergic conjunctivitis.

Dosing: One drop two times per day.

Considerations: Efficacy is not observed until 5–14 days of use.

H1-Antagonists

Similar to mast cell stabilizers, these topical medications are used for allergic conjunctivitis. Medications include bepotastine besilate (Bepreve Ophthalmic Solution®), epinastine hydrochloride (Elestat Ophthalmic Solution®), emedastine difumarate (Emadine Ophthalmic Solution®), alcaftadine (Lastacaft Ophthalmic Solution®), and azelastine hydrochloride (Optivar Ophthalmic Solution®).

Mechanism of action: These medications are H1-receptor antagonists.

Indications: Used for allergic conjunctivitis.

Dosing: One drop two times per day.

Considerations: Combination agents consisting of H1 antagonist-mast cell stabilizer ophthalmologic medications include olopatadine hydrochloride (Pataday Ophthalmic Solution®, Patanol Ophthalmic Solution®).

References

1. Nash EA, Margo CE. Patterns of emergency department visits for disorders of the eye and ocular adnexa. Arch Ophthalmol. 1998;116(9):1222–6.
2. Sklar DP, Lauth JE, Johnson DR. Topical anesthesia of the eye as a diagnostic test. Ann Emerg Med. 1989;18(11):1209–11.
3. Waldman N, Densie IK, Herbison P. Topical tetracaine used for 24 hours is safe and rated highly effective by patients for the treatment of pain caused by corneal abrasions: a double-blind, randomized clinical trial. Acad Emerg Med. 2014;21(4):374–82.
4. Swaminathan A, et al. The safety of topical anesthetics in the treatment of corneal abrasions: a review. J Emerg Med. 2015;49(5):810–5.
5. Puls HA, et al. Safety and effectiveness of topical anesthetics in corneal abrasions: systematic review and meta-analysis. J Emerg Med. 2015;49(5):816–24.
6. Walker RA, Adhikaris. Eye emergencies. In: Tintinalli's emergency medicine: a comprehensive study guide. 8th ed. Columbus: Mcgraw-Hill; 2016. Chap. 241.

7. Nizami RM. Treatment of ragweed allergic conjunctivitis with 2% cromolyn solution in unit doses. Ann Allergy. 1981;47:5.
8. Sharma R, Brunette DD. Ophthalmology. In: Rosen's emergency medicine. Philadelphia, PA: Saunders; 2014. p. 909–930.e2. Chapter 71.
9. http://www.aao.org/about/policies/color-codes-topical-ocular-medications.

Chapter 4
Eye Trauma

E. Liang Liu and Ashley Phipps

Brief Introduction

Ocular trauma is a common presentation to the emergency department in the United States, representing 3% of all ED visits every year [1] and remains the leading cause of monocular blindness [2]. Ocular trauma frequently follows assaults, workplace and sports injuries, and motor vehicle accidents. The trauma can range from a simple injury such as a superficial eyelid laceration to an ophthalmologic emergency such as a ruptured globe. The emergency physician must feel comfortable evaluating and managing these complaints, as trauma patients are at particular risk for vision-threatening injuries and increased morbidity [3].

Clinical Presentation

The diagnosis of ocular trauma requires a detailed history and specifically clarifying the mechanism of injury, especially whether it was blunt or penetrating. Penetrating injuries can

E. Liang Liu, MD (✉) · A. Phipps, MD
Department of Emergency Medicine, UT Southwestern Medical Center, Dallas, TX, USA

© Springer International Publishing AG, part of Springer Nature 2018

35

B. Long, A. Koyfman (eds.), *Handbook of Emergency Ophthalmology*, https://doi.org/10.1007/978-3-319-78945-3_4

cause minor injuries including eyelid lacerations, subconjunctival injuries, corneal abrasions or lacerations, traumatic iritis, and lens injuries to more complex injuries such as ruptured globes. Blunt trauma can result in corneal abrasions, hyphemas, traumatic mydriasis, lens dislocations, vitreous hemorrhages, retinal tears and detachments, traumatic iritis, choroidal ruptures, traumatic optic neuropathy, retrobulbar hemorrhages, and orbital blowout fractures in addition to globe ruptures.

Another approach to determining the injury involves identifying the part of the eye involved. This can be systematically evaluated by following the layers of the eye. The emergency physician should consider involvement of both intraorbital and extraorbital structures. Extraorbital structures include the eyelid, extraocular muscles, orbital bones, optic nerve, and brain. Intraorbital structures from outside include the conjunctiva, cornea, sclera, iris, anterior chamber, lens, posterior chamber, and retina.

A detailed eye examination is paramount to identifying the extent and severity of injuries. Where the history is lacking, the examination will also provide clues of the mechanism and structures of the eye involved. Particular caution should be taken in the polytrauma patient or patient with other facial injuries, as these injuries can distract from the ocular injury.

Differential Diagnosis

A number of both traumatic injuries and medical conditions can present concurrently. Depending on the mechanism, traumatic injuries usually do not isolate one specific part of the eye or involve just one pathology. An eyelid laceration can extend to involve the conjunctiva and deeper tissue to result in a ruptured globe. Subconjunctival hemorrhage, vitreous hemorrhage, and retrobulbar hemorrhage can occur independently but may also be found concurrently.

In considering ocular traumatic injury with a good mechanism, the physician should also consider the cause of the trauma and potential complications from the traumatic injury. The patient may have glaucoma, a corneal ulcer, or a burn that compromised their vision resulting in the accident. The eye examination may simply be a presentation of systemic disease. Patients may have a number of reasons to be at increased risk for infection and coagulopathy that may worsen an already vulnerable eye that has been injured.

This chapter will cover the following conditions:

1. Eyelid laceration
2. Conjunctival laceration
3. Corneal laceration
4. Traumatic hyphema
5. Iridodialysis/cyclodialysis
6. Ruptured globe
7. Orbital fracture
8. Retrobulbar hemorrhage
9. Intraocular foreign bodies
10. Chemical burn

Clinical Evaluation

History

There are several features of the history that are important when evaluating for ocular trauma. As mentioned above, one of most important historical features for ocular trauma is what the exact mechanism of injury is. Generally speaking, any suspicion for a penetrating or perforating eye injury requires prompt evaluation and definitive management. If a projectile was involved, the size, type, and velocity of the projectile are important predictors of severity of damage, as small high-velocity projectiles increase the risk for a penetrating injury, whereas a larger object is more likely to result in blunt injury such as a fracture of the orbital wall [4].

The use of eye protection can help the clinician decide the likelihood of injury and extent of potential injury. However, penetrating eye injuries can occur even with eye protection in place. It is also necessary to know exactly when the trauma occurred and when symptoms started to understand progression of injury and establish an accurate timeline. For example, an injury that just occurred would be less likely to present with secondary sequelae such as infection and mass effect from hemorrhage, compared to one that is several hours to days old. Any history of previous trauma or surgery is also important as any previous compromise to the structural integrity of the eye can increase risk for reinjury.

Characterizing the patient's symptoms after the trauma is essential including:

1. Is there pain or eye discomfort such as a scratchiness or foreign body feeling?

   (a). Does anything make the pain better or worse?
   (b). Is there change in pain at rest or on movement?

2. Is there associated photophobia?
3. Is there any change in vision including loss of vision, blurred vision, or double vision?
4. Are there any associated non-ocular injuries?

As in any patient with trauma, it is also beneficial to review the patient's past medical history. If there are any concerns of abrasions, lacerations, or penetrating injury, the patient's last known tetanus immunization should be documented and tetanus vaccine provided if indicated [5].

Physical Examination

A focused ocular physical examination as described in the previous chapters is required in all patients presenting with ocular trauma and can frequently determine the diagnosis without further testing.

1. *General inspection*: If the eyelids are swollen shut, avoid putting pressure on the orbit in an attempt to pry the eyelids open. Instead, insert a bent paperclip or commercial eyelid retractor under both lids to open the eyelids [5].

   (a). How does the eye and orbit look on gross examination? Is there any periorbital edema, ecchymosis, or lacerations?
   (b). Are any facial fractures noted?
   (c). How does the orbit look—Is there any proptosis? Does the orbit itself look flat compared to the other eye? If the eye looks flat, a ruptured globe is suspected, and the examination can stop here with placement of an eye shield and emergent ophthalmology consultation [5]. See the section below for further management of a ruptured globe.
   (d). Any foreign body hidden underneath the upper eyelid?
   (e). What about the pupils—Are they irregular or teardrop? Are they equal and reactive? Is there a relative afferent pupillary defect as may be noted in the setting of a retinal detachment, vitreous hemorrhage, or retrobulbar hemorrhage?
   (f). Is there a hyphema present?

2. *Visual acuity*: Typically this will be decreased, but it is important to determine whether a decrease is due to clouding, dryness of the eye, or intraocular cause.

3. *Extraocular movements*: This is especially important in trauma to assess as reduced extraocular movements can suggest a ruptured globe, orbital wall fracture with entrapment of the extraocular muscles, nerve palsy, or retrobulbar hematoma. If the eyelids are too swollen and the patient is unable to open the eye, bedside ultrasound can aid in the extraocular movement exam.

4. *Fluorescein testing*: This stain helps to evaluate for epithelial defects as well as test for a Seidel's sign. The Seidel's test is used to detect difficult to visualize corneal injuries that allows leaking of aqueous humor from the anterior

chamber. The fluorescein dye is applied to the eye over the site of injury, with particular attention paid to the region of the suspected laceration. The test is positive when a stream of fluorescent dye is visualized from the site of injury on slit lamp examination. While specific, a negative test does not rule out a full thickness corneal laceration. This is extremely important to do prior to evaluating the intraocular pressure. If there is a positive Seidel's sign, the patient has a ruptured globe until proven otherwise. Again, put a protective covering over the eye and do not test intraocular pressures.

5. *Tonometry*: Use tonometry to test the intraocular pressure in those without concern for open globe. This can help aid in the diagnosis of retrobulbar hematoma and secondary glaucoma among other conditions.

6. *Slit lamp exam*: Oftentimes the slit lamp exam can reveal defects and irregularities that are difficult to visualize with the naked eye. Examine the eyelid including everting the lid to search for concealed laceration or potential foreign bodies. Examine the cornea for any foreign bodies and also determine if a rust ring can be visualized. Look for defects in the cornea or sclera or distortion of the anterior chamber structures such as a shallow anterior chamber or a hyphema. In blunt trauma, rupture can be seen at the limbus. Additionally, cell and flare can be seen on slit lamp with cases of traumatic iritis [5].

7. *Fundoscopy*: On fundoscopy, the red reflex may be abnormal, suggesting a defect in the lens, cornea, anterior chamber, posterior chamber, or retina. Retinal injuries, vitreous hemorrhage, and potential foreign bodies can also be seen on fundoscopy.

8. *Ocular ultrasound*: Especially in patients who refuse to open their eyes due to photophobia or pain, bedside ultrasound is an extension of the physical examination that can provide information necessary for diagnosis. By applying sufficient lubricating gel, the eye can be protected from the examination in the case of a ruptured globe. Ultrasound can

reveal hemorrhage, distortion to the globe, abnormalities in the anterior and posterior chambers, retinal detachment, retrobulbar hematoma, lens subluxation or dislocation, presence of an intraocular foreign body, defects to the optic nerve, and other pathology.

Clinical Conditions and Management

Though management will depend on the pathology, some general principles of management are common among traumatic ocular injuries. The first step of management is to protect the eye to prevent further injury which may require placement of an eye shield. Antibiotics should be given and tetanus vaccine updated to avoid complications of infection and tetanus. Supportive care including analgesia and antiemetics are required. If open globe is suspected or confirmed, the patient needs bed rest and supportive measures to minimize increases in intraocular pressure. While follow-up with ophthalmology is recommended for any eye injury, only a handful of conditions require immediate consultation (Table 4.1).

TABLE 4.1 Ophthalmology follow-up for traumatic injury

Immediate consultation	24-h follow-up
Chemical burns of the eye	Anterior hyphema
Perforation of the globe or cornea	Blowout fracture
Lens dislocation	Retinal injuries
Retrobulbar hemorrhage with increased intraocular pressure	
Lacerations involving the lid margin, tarsal plate, or nasolacrimal drainage system	
Optic nerve injury	

Eyelid Laceration

The eyelids are the first level of protection to the eyes, and injuries to the eyelid can significantly impact the underlying eye. The eyelid's role is to keep the eyes moist and protected from foreign bodies. Thus, an injured eyelid can result in eye dryness and irritation, as well as increasing the risk for infection and further injury. Eyelid injuries result in significant swelling to the lid itself. Both penetrating and blunt trauma can cause an eyelid laceration. Blunt trauma to the cheek or zygoma may be associated with an avulsion of the medial canthus and a canalicular laceration. It is important to evaluate the laceration and ensure it does not involve the lacrimal duct system or the orbit. The eyelids should always be fully everted to evaluate for deeper extension. The examination should also include assessment of the extraocular muscles, as they can be commonly injured. If ptosis or orbital fat is visible on inspection, the laceration may extend through the orbital septum, indicating a deeper laceration with increased risk for infection. Evaluation for foreign body and globe injury should also be performed via examination and potentially imaging as needed [5, 6].

Emergency physicians should feel comfortable performing laceration repair on all partial thickness lid lacerations other than those affecting the lacrimal system or lid margin. 6-0 nylon sutures should be used and removed within 5 days [1]. Any laceration that is within 8 mm of the medial canthus should be evaluated for lacrimal system involvement. As the lacrimal ducts are important for proper drainage of tears, lacrimal duct injuries require repair by an ophthalmologist and, if not treated appropriately, can cause significant morbidity. Lacerations involving the lid margin will often require repair by ophthalmology, as any notching of the lid may lead to improper closure of the eyelids and long-term sequelae [5, 6].

Conjunctival Laceration

Patients with traumatic conjunctival lacerations will often be asymptomatic, as the conjunctiva is poorly innervated and vision is rarely affected. If symptomatic, the patient may complain of pain, tearing, or foreign body sensation. Fluorescein staining of the conjunctiva and evaluation with slit lamp is essential to evaluate for an open globe and to identify the laceration. Management of conjunctival laceration depends on the depth and extent of the injury. Lacerations smaller than 1–1.5 cm in length generally heal spontaneously without intervention. However, if the conjunctiva is not well approximated or folded over, realignment may be needed. Larger lacerations require repair by an ophthalmologist. Follow-up after repair should be within 1 week of the injury for large lacerations and can be as needed for smaller lacerations. All of these patients should be given a topical antibiotic ointment such as erythromycin or bacitracin/polymyxin B [5, 6].

Corneal Laceration

In contrast to the conjunctiva, the cornea is richly innervated. Corneal pathology including laceration may result in exquisite pain and associated decrease in vision. If a corneal laceration is suspected, fluorescein staining and a slit lamp examination should be performed. If the anterior chamber appears shallow compared to the unaffected eye or there is a positive Seidel test, a full thickness corneal laceration is present, equivalent to a ruptured globe. The eye should be immediately covered with an eye shield and ophthalmology consulted. If there is no ruptured globe, the patient may have a partial thickness corneal laceration. These patients can be sent home with 24-h follow-up with ophthalmology, cycloplegic eye drops such as scopolamine, and a topical antibiotic [5, 6].

Traumatic Hyphema

Traumatic hyphema occurs when blood enters the anterior chamber typically due to a blunt injury of the eye. The majority of cases occur in males, with 60% related to sports injury [7]. Hyphemas are usually self-limited but can result in further ocular complications such as obstructing aqueous outflow of the anterior chamber resulting in increased intraocular pressures. Approximately one third of patients with a traumatic hyphema have an elevated intraocular pressure [8]. There is also risk for rebleed within 10 days which can result in secondary glaucoma, corneal blood staining, and damage to the optic nerve [4]. Typically, patients with hyphema will have immediate visual compromise at the time of injury. Examination consists of determining the size of the hyphema, the location of the blood, and intraocular pressure measurement. An ultrasound can be helpful if the fundus cannot be viewed, and a CT may be necessary to evaluate for a foreign body. In the patient with frequent hyphemas or minimal mechanism of injury, coagulopathy, sickle cell disease, and anticoagulant use should be considered on the differential.

Hospitalization is required in the setting of high intraocular pressures, hyphema involving greater than 50% of the anterior chamber, and in the pediatric population, given its risk of causing irreversible amblyopia [4, 7]. General management with uncomplicated hyphema includes restriction of activities and minimizing risk of reinjury. Administration of a cycloplegic (atropine) and corticosteroid eye drops with patching of the affected eye have also been recommended, but additional studies also suggest that perhaps these interventions have no additional benefit [4]. In the setting of increased intraocular pressure, topical and systemic ocular hypertension medications including timolol and oral carbonic anhydrase inhibitors can be helpful. Surgical management may be necessary to reduce intraocular pressures. Some studies have indicated antifibrinolytic agents such as aminocaproic acid and tranexamic acid may be beneficial, especially in the prevention of secondary hemorrhage [9, 10].

Iridodialysis/Cyclodialysis

Iridodialysis is when a portion of the iris becomes disconnected from the ciliary body, while cyclodialysis is when the actual ciliary body becomes detached from the sclera (Fig. 4.1). These patients will often be asymptomatic but can

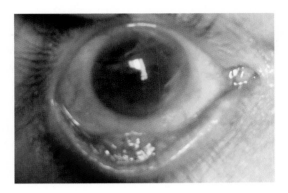

FIGURE 4.1 Traumatic iridodialysis in a patient hit by a rock in the eye while landscaping

have vision changes such as diplopia or photophobia. Iridodialysis is sometimes referred to as the development of a "secondary pupil," as the resulting iris defect will make the eye look like there are two pupils. These injuries often times have a concomitant hyphema [1]. The primary complication is elevated intraocular pressure resulting in acute glaucoma. Urgent follow-up with ophthalmology is required [6].

Ruptured Globe

A ruptured globe can occur with penetrating and blunt trauma. Patients will present with decreased vision and eye pain. Exam findings can include an irregular or peaked pupil, hyphema, subconjunctival hemorrhage or chemosis, flat or deep anterior chamber compared to the unaffected eye, dislocated lens, or new cataract. If a ruptured globe is suspected, avoid any pressure on the eye and cover it with an eye shield immediately. Fluorescein staining can be completed to evaluate for Seidel's sign. A CT scan of the brain and orbits should be performed with 1 mm sections to evaluate for the ruptured globe as well as any intraocular foreign body. An emergent ophthalmology consultation is needed. Patients should be made NPO, placed on bedrest, and told to avoid straining (Valsalva, bending over) to avoid increasing the intraocular pressure. Antiemetics should be given as needed to prevent vomiting, as again this increases intraocular pressure. Systemic intravenous antibiotics should be started immediately. In adults, cefazolin or vancomycin in addition to ciprofloxacin is recommended, while in children, cefazolin and gentamicin are recommended. All patients need to receive tetanus prophylaxis if greater than 5 years since their previous vaccination, as well as pain medications as needed [5, 6, 11].

Orbital Fracture

Orbital fractures typically occur due to blunt trauma. Signs and symptoms can include pain especially with eye movement, inability to move the eye in a certain direction, diplopia, and crepitus after nose blowing. The most common orbital fractures are orbital floor through the maxillary sinus and medial wall through the ethmoid sinus. With an orbital floor fracture, the patient may complain of pain and difficulty with upward gaze secondary to entrapment of the inferior rectus muscle. A medial wall fracture may cause complaints of pain and difficulty looking side to side. Sensation loss inferior to the eye and ipsilateral nose often indicates an inferior orbital sensory nerve injury.

Plain radiographs of the skull are rarely used for detecting orbital fractures. Several studies have shown a poor sensitivity of 64–78% for detecting orbital fractures on plain films. A CT scan of the orbits is the gold standard for detecting orbital fractures, with increased sensitivity of 79–96% [1]. Patients with an orbital fracture and entrapment, or those exhibiting signs of the oculocardiac reflex (bradycardia, heart block, syncope), need urgent follow-up with ophthalmology within 24 h for surgical repair. All other patients can be discharged home with follow-up within 1–2 weeks. Patients should be instructed to avoid blowing their nose and use ice packs as needed for pain and swelling. In immunocompromised patients or uncontrolled diabetics, consider a week course of oral antibiotics such as cephalexin, erythromycin, or doxycycline [5, 6].

Retrobulbar Hemorrhage

Retrobulbar hemorrhage typically occurs after significant blunt trauma. Patients will present with decreased vision and also have significant associated periorbital swelling and ecchymosis. The eye may look proptotic with tense eyelids that are very hard to open, chemosis, and subconjunctival hemorrhage. If the hemorrhage is significant, orbital compartment syndrome can develop, as the orbit is a relatively enclosed space surrounded by bony walls and an inflexible orbital septum [1]. This increase in pressure can compress the optic nerve leading to ischemia. If not recognized quickly, within 90 min of ischemia, the nerve damage can become permanent. After evaluation for open globe with fluorescein staining and ensuring its absence, intraocular pressure should be measured. If there is evidence of optic neuropathy such as a dilated or nonreactive pupil or the intraocular pressure is greater than 40 mmHg, an immediate lateral canthotomy and cantholysis should be performed [5, 6].

Intraocular Foreign Bodies

Intraocular foreign bodies can often be seen with metal workers or welders, with up to 80% of cases occurring with hammering [1]. Generally the patient has a history of some eye trauma or with the feeling that an object hit the eye. Usually these patients have pain or foreign body sensation and photophobia, and they may have vision changes. Certain metals such as iron, steel, tin, and copper as well as organic material can cause significant inflammation. Bedside ultrasonography or a CT scan of the orbits can be used to evaluate for an intraocular foreign body. However, it is important to remember that some organic material will not be seen on CT scan [1]. Consider a ruptured or open globe which is often associated with this injury. If an intraocular foreign body is found, discuss with ophthalmology. Most patients will require antibiotics and urgent surgical removal to prevent infection. If the decision is made to not remove the intraocular foreign body, close ophthalmology follow-up is needed for serial exams to evaluate for delayed inflammation or infection requiring intervention [6].

Chemical Burn

Chemical burns are ocular emergencies and require copious irrigation immediately, unless a ruptured globe is suspected. Irrigation is recommended continuously for 30 min with normal saline or lactated ringers. This can be facilitated with the use of topical anesthetic and an eye speculum to hold the eye open. It is important to ensure the lids are everted and the entire surface is irrigated. Never attempt to neutralize an alkali burn by instilling an acid or vice versa, as this can lead to further harm. After irrigation, wait 10 min and then check the pH using litmus paper. Irrigation is repeated until the pH is between 7 and 7.4. A moistened cotton-tipped applicator can be used to remove any material from the conjunctival fornices. Also determine the type and time of exposure. Alkali injuries are more common, as alkaline substances are frequently present in household products such as lye, ammonia, drain cleaners, and fertilizers [12]. Alkaline substance causes liquefactive necrosis which can penetrate deep into the tissue, while acids cause coagulation necrosis which rarely penetrates deeply into the tissue [5, 6, 11].

After irrigation, the eye should then be fully examined looking for any conjunctival blanching, chemosis, hemorrhages, and corneal opacification. Fluorescein staining can help evaluate for an epithelial defect, and intraocular pressure should always be measured to evaluate for swelling due to the chemical burn. These patients all need urgent ophthalmology follow-up within 24 h. They can generally be discharged with topical antibiotic ointment, pain medication, frequent preservative-free artificial tears while awake, and cycloplegic drops. If the burn is severe, topical steroid drops may also be prescribed [5, 6, 11]. However, prescription of topical steroid drops should only be done in association with an ophthalmologist.

Disposition

Complications of ocular trauma include permanent loss of vision, corneal ulcers that may lead to delayed perforation, infection especially endophthalmitis, and sympathetic ophthalmia. Sympathetic ophthalmia is an autoimmune-mediated response to the uninjured eye that occurs weeks to months after the initial injury. This can occur if enucleation of the severely traumatized eye is not performed initially or within 1–2 weeks after severe damage, as the uveal tissue that is typically sequestered becomes exposed with injury. Patients present with pain, photophobia, and decreased visual acuity. Management requires ophthalmology evaluation and typically treatment with steroids and immunosuppressants.

Pearls/Pitfalls

- If a ruptured globe is considered, immediately place an eye shield and consult ophthalmology.
- Most traumatic eye injuries can be properly treated in the emergency room and discharged home with urgent ophthalmology follow-up.
- Don't forget to think of other associated injuries that may have occurred with the trauma such as intracranial or cervical spine injuries.
- Wearing eye protection does not prevent injury but can significantly reduce it.

References

1. Bord SP, Linden J. Trauma to the globe and orbit. Emerg Med Clin North Am. 2008;26(1):97–123.
2. McGwin G, Owsley C. Incidence of emergency department – treated eye injury in the United States. Arch Ophthalmol. 2005;123(5):662–6.
3. Kim G, Wong MM. Ocular trauma: an evidence-based approach to evaluation and management in the ED. Pediatr Emerg

Med Pract. 2006;3(11):1–15. https://www.ebmedicine.net/topics. php?paction=showTopic&topic_id=180.

4. Güzel M, Erenler AK, Niyaz L, Baydın A. Management of traumatic eye injuries in the emergency department. OA Emerg Med. 2014;2(1):2.

5. Tintinalli JE, et al. Eye emergencies. In: Tintinalli's emergency medicine: a comprehensive study guide. New York: McGraw-Hill; 2011. p. 7.

6. Gerstenblith AT, Rabinowitz MP. The wills eye manual: office and emergency room diagnosis and treatment of eye disease. 6th ed. Philadelphia, PA: Lippincott Williams & Wilkins; 2012.

7. Gharaibeh A, Savage HI, Scherer RW, Goldberg MF, Lindsley K. Medical interventions for traumatic hyphema. Cochrane Database Syst Rev. 2013;12:CD005431.

8. Walton W, Von Hagen S, Grigorian R, Zarbin M. Management of traumatic hyphema. Surv Ophthalmol. 2002;47(4):297–334.

9. Crouch ER Jr, Williams PB, Gray MK, et al. Topical amino-caproic acid in the treatment of traumatic hyphema. Arch Ophthalmol. 1997;115:1106–12.

10. Romano PE, Robinson JA. Traumatic hyphema: a comprehensive review of the past half century yields 8076 cases for which specific medical treatment reduces rebleeding 62%, from 13% to 5% (p_.0001). Binocul Vis Strabismus Q. 2000;15:175–86.

11. Stone CK, Humphries RL. Eye emergencies. In: Current diagnosis & treatment emergency medicine. 7th ed. New York: McGraw-Hill; 2011.

12. Naradzay J, Barish RA. Approach to ophthalmologic emergencies. Med Clin North Am. 2006;90(2):305–28.

Chapter 5
Eyelid Disorders

Matthew Streitz

Brief Introduction

Eye complaints account for approximately 1–2% of all ED visits. Eye emergencies can be categorized into three categories: the red eye, the painful eye, and those with associated vision loss. This chapter will focus mainly on the eyelid and common disorders emergency physicians need to be able to diagnose and treat upon their presentation. This chapter will discuss the presentation, evaluation, treatment, and disposition for stye, chalazion, blepharitis, dacryocystitis, and ectropion.

Clinical Presentation

Those presenting to the ED with eye-related concerns present in a myriad of ways, just like every other chief complaint. The job of the emergency physician is to rule out the life, limb, or eyesight threats. Common patient complaints are double vision, redness, pain, foreign body sensation or foreign

M. Streitz, MD
Department of Emergency Medicine, San Antonio Uniformed Services Health Education Consortium, San Antonio, TX, USA

© Springer International Publishing AG, part of Springer Nature 2018
B. Long, A. Koyfman (eds.), *Handbook of Emergency Ophthalmology*, https://doi.org/10.1007/978-3-319-78945-3_5

51

body in the eye, vision loss, color vision changes, floaters, and a "dark curtain," as well as redness, tenderness, or swelling of the structures around the eye.

Stye (hordeolum): An acute infection (typically staphylococcal), which involves the sebaceous secretions in the glands of Zeis (*external hordeolum*, or *stye*) or the meibomian glands (*internal hordeolum*) in the tarsal plate [1] (Fig. 5.1). Patients typically present with a localized painful swelling of one or both eyelids. Commonly the chief complaint can be a "generalized swelling or erythema" of the lid which does not become localized until later in the course. It is also common to have a history of either a stye or chalazia upon further history. Hordeolum can be either internal or external. External hordeolum infections often appear to center around an eyelash follicle. The natural progression is to develop over a few days, resolving spontaneously a few short days later. Although uncommon, superficial cellulitis or even an abscess may develop from a persistent hordeolum. In such cases, systemic antibiotic therapy and possible surgical incision and drainage may be required. Hordeola and subsequently chalazia are found more frequently in patients with a history of dry eyes and chronic blepharitis [1, 2].

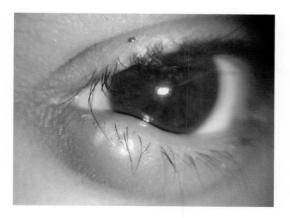

FIGURE 5.1 External Stye, obtained from Wikipedia, 11 Jan 2018

Chalazion: This results from chronic granulomatous inflammation, typically of an obstructed meibomian gland from an unresolved internal hordeolum (Fig. 5.2). If chalazia are left untreated, they can continue to grow, and large chalazia can cause secondary visual complications leading to induced astigmatism (corneal distortion) or reduction of the peripheral visual fields. Although rare, cellulitis of the eyelid may occur if an internal hordeolum is untreated and becomes chronic. Most morbidity associated with chalazia is secondary to improper drainage of the inflamed tissue.

Blepharitis: A condition with chronic eyelid inflammation of the meibomian glands that affects upward of 37–47% of patients seen by ophthalmology [3] (Fig. 5.3). It is associated with acute exacerbations and other dermatologic conditions like seborrheic dermatitis and rosacea. The likely bacterium involved in acute exacerbations is *S. epidermis*, accounting for roughly 50% of cases. Blepharitis can either be anterior or posterior. Anterior affects the eyelid skin, base of the eyelashes, and the eyelash follicles and can be further be subdivided into staphylococcal or seborrheic blepharitis. Posterior blepharitis affects the meibomian glands, and the major cause is secondary to meibomian gland dysfunction (MGD) [2–6]. Patient demographics include all ethnic groups equally and women at a 4:1 ratio. Although all ages can present with blepharitis, the mean age is 42 years old.

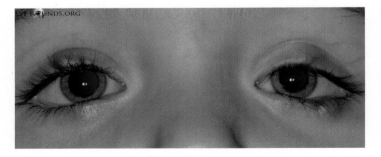

FIGURE 5.2 Chalazion, obtained from EyeRounds.org, 11 Jan 2018

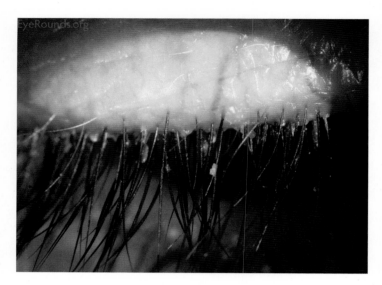

FIGURE 5.3 Blepharitis, obtained from EyeRounds.org, 17 Jan 2017

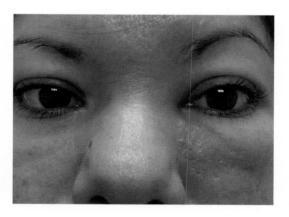

FIGURE 5.4 Dacryocystitis, obtained with patient permission

Dacryocystitis: A bacterial infection of the lacrimal sac commonly is caused by *S. aureus*, *S. epidermis*, and alpha- and beta-hemolytic strep (Fig. 5.4). The infection is frequently due to nasolacrimal duct obstruction and presents in a bimodal distribution of infants and adults over 40 years old. There is a slight female predominance to this condition due to a narrow duct diameter [2, 5, 7, 8]. When present in the neonatal period, this is a condition with a potential for significant morbidity and mortality due to the poorly developed orbital septum. This can lead to brain abscesses, meningitis, sepsis, and death as possible complications. Prompt diagnosis and treatment are vital.

Ectropion: Ectropion is a condition involving the lower lid, and on presentation the lid is turned outward (Figs. 5.5 and 5.6). There are typically three main causes/types: involutional, or an increased horizontal laxity to the lid; cicatricial, where a shortening of the anterior lamella due to scarring causes the outward turn; and finally paralytic, which occurs as the tone of the orbicularis muscle supporting the lower eyelid is lost. Paralytic is most commonly secondary to a facial nerve palsy.

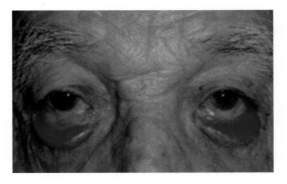

FIGURE 5.5 Ectropion, obtained from omicsonline.org, 18 Jan 2017

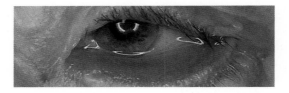

FIGURE 5.6 Ectropion, obtained from omicsonline.org, 18 Jan 2017

Other types, although much more rare, are congenital and mechanical. Mechanical is due to a mass effect or displacement secondary to a tumor or mass.

Differential Diagnosis

There is a broad differential diagnosis for eyelid disorders because redness, swelling, or tenderness of the eyelid does not exclude other pathology that may be more concerning. The differential for those complaints includes cellulitis (septal and preseptal), dacryocystitis, chalazion, hordeolum (stye), dacryoadenitis, anaphylaxis, conjunctivitis, keratitis, and endophthalmitis. Other, more specific eyelid diagnoses are cyst, carcinoma, xanthelasma, papilloma, pyogenic granuloma, amyloid deposition, and any skin condition that can be found elsewhere on the body can be found on the eyelid [4, 9]. This chapter will discuss chalazion, stye, blepharitis, dacryocystitis, and ectropion, but in doing so the large differential must be remembered during the evaluation.

Evaluation

A solid understanding of the anatomy of the eye and the surrounding structures provides a good foundation for working up and diagnosing any eye complaint. This has been discussed in Chap. 2. The specific evaluation and physical examination findings for the specific conditions are as follows:

Stye (hordeolum): Erythematous and tender eyelid nodule with possible purulent material released from the outer eyelash line is present in external hordeola. With internal hordeola, purulent material may be released on the conjunctival surface of eyelid (Fig. 5.1).

Chalazion: Typical examination findings are a hard, rubbery, painless nodule along the lid margin (Fig. 5.2).

Blepharitis: Bilateral red and dry eyes, gritty foreign body or burning sensation, crusting of eyelashes, blurry vision, tearing, and sometimes photophobia are common. If the cause is secondary to seborrheic dermatitis, there is likely to be more of an oily appearance to the eyelash and less erythema on examination. Symptoms are typically worse in the morning. Staphylococcal blepharitis may also present with missing eyelashes or eyelashes that are out of alignment with surrounding eyelashes and is classically found with no other forms (Fig. 5.3).

Dacryocystitis: Erythema, swelling, and tenderness along the lacrimal sac are present. Severe infections can present with sepsis and other systemic signs of illness. Pressure over the area of fluctuance may produce purulent discharge from the puncta. In an acute presentation, the sac may rupture and a fistula may form, frequently closing a few days after the onset [8]. Drainage from the site is common until the lesion closes. Look for signs of preseptal cellulitis, meningitis, abscess, and sepsis (Fig. 5.4).

Ectropion: An outward turning of the lower eyelid is present. Patients present with tearing, grittiness or irritation, and red eyes. Symptoms are a result of inadequate lubrication and closure of the eyelid margins (Figs. 5.5 and 5.6).

Management

Chalazia and hordeola may be treated by applying warm compresses to the eyelid several times per day (15 min four times a day), helping to accelerate drainage of the lesion. In some cases, one or multiple eyelashes can be plucked to promote drainage. In the event of a stye, antibiotic ointments such as erythromycin ophthalmic ointment for 7–10 days with concomitant steroid use may help a stye to resolve more rapidly. Acute chalazion can be treated with the same antibiotic ointment as a stye with the addition of a 14–21-day regimen of doxycycline (100 mg BID for adults and 2.2 mg/kg/dose BID for children) [10, 11] (Table 5.1). If superficial cellulitis or abscess develops from a persistent hordeola/chalazia, systemic antibiotic therapy coupled with possible surgical incision and drainage may be required.

TABLE 5.1 Treatment recommendations

Condition	Symptomatic treatment	Medication treatments	
Stye (hordeolum)	Warm compresses (15 min QID)	Erythromycin ophthalmic ointment	
Chalazion	Warm compresses (15 min QID)	Acute: Erythromycin ophthalmic ointment Acute on chronic: Doxycycline 100 mg BID for 14–21 days (2.2 mg/kg per dose BID for children)	Cellulitis/abscess: 1. Systemic antibiotics 2. Surgical drainage
Blepharitis	Warm compresses (15 min QID) Scrub eyelid margin (mild soap/shampoo) Artificial tears	*Topical*: 1. Bacitracin BID 2–8 weeks 2. Erythromycin ophthalmic ointment BID for 2–8 weeks *Systemic (not responding to topical) Tetracyclines*: 1. Tetracycline 100 mg daily 2. Doxycycline 100 mg daily 3. Minocycline 100 mg daily – Continue until ophthalmology follow-up *Macrolides*: 1. Erythromycin 250–500 mg daily 2. Azithromycin 250–500 mg daily or 1 g weekly × 3 weeks – Continue until ophthalmology follow-up Corticosteroid drops Cyclosporine TID or QID may be helpful *Combination (steroid/antibiotic) drops*: 1. Tobramycin/dexamethasone 2. Tobramycin/loteprednol	

TABLE 5.1 (continued)

Condition	Symptomatic treatment	Medication treatments
Dacryocystitis	Warm compresses (15 min QID) Gentle massage	*Mild to moderate infections*: 1. Erythromycin ophthalmic ointment 2. Oral antibiotics—augmentin, clindamycin, and cephalexin Severe cases (abscess formation, meningitis, or sepsis) require urgent intravenous antibiotics 1. Vancomycin 2. Third-generation cephalosporin
Ectropion	Lubricating agents (erythromycin ophthalmic ointment)	

Blepharitis: Treatment consists of applying warm compresses to the eyelid several times per day (15 min four times a day) in addition to scrubbing the lid margin with mild soap/shampoo and a washcloth. Artificial tears may also provide symptomatic relief. Cultures of the eyelid margins may be helpful for follow-up with ophthalmology and for those patients with recurrent infection or evidence of severe inflammation. Confirming diagnosis is typically out of the scope of the ED. Antibiotic choices for blepharitis include topical agents like bacitracin and erythromycin applied to the margins of the eyelids twice daily for 2–8 weeks (Table 5.1). For those patients not responding to topical agents, oral antibiotics such as tetracycline, doxycycline, and minocycline are options [2–5, 10, 11]. Finally, steroids have been shown to have a small benefit for patients with significant evidence of inflammation along the eyelid margins. Corticosteroid drops three to four times daily, cyclosporine, or combination drugs like tobramycin/dexamethasone or tobramycin/loteprednol have also shown promise in treating infection/inflammation.

In addition, steroid ointments can be applied until inflammation has subsided. Patients should always be made aware of the potential side effects of tetracycline antibiotics such as photosensitization and GI upset. For steroids, these include elevated intraocular pressure and cataracts.

Dacryocystitis: Warm compresses and gentle massage will express purulent material. Mild to moderate infections can be managed using topical (erythromycin ointment) and oral antibiotics—augmentin, clindamycin, and cephalexin with outpatient ophthalmology referral (Table 5.1). Severe cases such as those with abscess formation, meningitis, or sepsis require urgent ophthalmology referral, admission with intravenous antibiotics, and likely percutaneous drainage [8]. Antibiotics should cover methicillin-resistant *Staphylococcus aureus* (MRSA) and typically include vancomycin and a third-generation cephalosporin.

Ectropion: Definitive management of the condition is surgical. Medical management is temporizing until surgery can take place and includes lubricating agents.

Disposition

Chalazion and stye: Routine follow-up with an ophthalmologist is necessary to monitor and document resolution and to monitor for side effects from medications. In the event the lesions do not resolve, surgical drainage may be warranted.

Blepharitis: Discharge to home with ophthalmology referral is appropriate with appropriate antibiotics; topical versus oral with the addition of steroids through coordination with ophthalmology.

Dacryocystitis: In patients who are well-appearing and in whom follow-up can be confirmed, discharge to home is appropriate where those with significant involvement, poor ability to follow-up, or concerns for the major complications of dacryocystitis require inpatient treatment with ophthalmology.

Ectropion: Discharge home with lubricating agents and a referral to an ophthalmologist is appropriate.

Pearls/Pitfalls

An incomplete physical examination, particularly a visual acuity with the addition of a slit lamp examination would potentially be a major pitfall with treatment of the above conditions. Other pitfalls are not adequately covering for the likely bacteria responsible for each condition and inadequate or untimely ophthalmology referral and evaluation.

References

1. Kumar V, Robbins SL. Robbins basic pathology. 8th ed. Philadelphia, PA: Saunders/Elsevier; 2007.
2. American Academy of Ophthalmology. Preferred practice pattern: blepharitis. October 2012 revision. https://www.aao.org/preferred-practice-pattern/blepharitis-ppp--2013. Accessed 10 Nov 2016.
3. Lemp MA, Nichols KK. Blepharitis in the United States 2009: a survey-based perspective on prevalence and treatment. Ocul Surf. 2009;7(Suppl 2):S1–14.
4. Lindsley K, Matsumura S, Hatef E, Akpek EK. Interventions for chronic blepharitis. Cochrane Database Syst Rev. 2012;5:CD005556.
5. Pflugfelder SC, Karpecki PM, Perez VL. Treatment of blepharitis: recent clinical trials. Ocul Surf. 2014;12(4):273–84.
6. Perry HD, Doshi-Carnevale S, Donnenfeld ED, et al. Efficacy of commercially available topical cyclosporine A 0.05% in the treatment of meibomian gland dysfunction. Cornea. 2006;25:171–5.
7. Skuta GL, Cantor LB, Cioffi GA, et al., editors. American Academy of Ophthalmology basic clinical science course: external disease and cornea. Vol. 8. San Francisco, CA: American Academy of Ophthalmology; 2013. p. 44–50. 58–66.
8. Pinar-Sueiro S, Sota M, Lerchundi TX, Gibelalde A, Berasategui B, Vilar B, Hernandez JL. Dacryocystitis: systematic approach to diagnosis and therapy. Curr Infect Dis Rep. 2012;14(2):137–46.
9. Kanski JJ, Bowling B. Clinical ophthalmology: a systemic approach. 7th ed. New York: Elsevier Saunders; 2011. p. 34–9.

10. Marx JA, Rosen P. Rosen's emergency medicine: concepts and clinical practice. 8th ed. Philadelphia, PA: Elsevier/Saunders; 2014. Chapter 71.
11. Tintinalli JE, Stapczynski JS, Ma OJ, Yealy DM, Meckler GD, Cline D. Tintinalli's emergency medicine: a comprehensive study guide. 8th ed. New York: McGraw-Hill Education; 2016. Chapter 241.

Chapter 6
Evaluation of the Red Eye

Paul Basel

Brief Introduction

The red eye is a common complaint in the emergency department. While the majority of these visits will be for benign causes, the role of the emergency physician is to appropriately evaluate for vision-threatening complaints.

Differential Diagnosis

The differential diagnosis for the red eye is wide and includes chemical and radiation exposures, infectious, traumatic, allergic, and autoimmune causes. Patients usually present with symptoms in addition to discoloration of the eye.

P. Basel, MD
Department of Emergency Medicine, San Antonio Uniformed Services Health Education Consortium, San Antonio, TX, USA

© Springer International Publishing AG, part of Springer Nature 2018
B. Long, A. Koyfman (eds.), *Handbook of Emergency Ophthalmology*, https://doi.org/10.1007/978-3-319-78945-3_6

Evaluation

History

A thorough history is essential and will help narrow your differential. History should include:

- History of contact lens use. If positive, question about type, hygiene, and frequency of changing
- Timing of symptoms
- Systemic symptoms (fever, rashes, upper respiratory symptoms, etc.)
- Recent infections
- Characterization of symptoms (pain, burning, etc.)
- Visual changes
- Occupational and recreational exposures
- History of prior symptoms
- Contacts with similar symptoms
- Recent travel
- Past medical history especially:
  - Prior ocular complaints and surgeries
  - Autoimmune disorders
  - Immunosuppressive disorders
  - Diabetes
- Family history of autoimmune diseases
- Complete medication list focusing on new medications, immunosuppressive medications, and any history of topical corticosteroid use

Physical Examination

A thorough physical examination for ocular complaints includes the following:

1. Visual acuity—Compare bilateral exam and to patient's baseline, if known. If the patient uses corrective lens at baseline, allow use during exam, or provide a pinhole occluder for accurate testing.

2. General appearance—Note conjunctiva injection, edema, chemosis, subconjunctival hemorrhages, etc. Note any signs or trauma. Complete a thorough physical examination looking for signs of systemic disease (rashes, cough, congestion, etc.).
3. Pupil exam—Note pupil size and reactivity. Evaluate for consensual photophobia and afferent pupillary defect.
4. Intraocular pressures—Bilateral ocular pressures should be obtained in most situations. If there is concern for open globe based on history and general appearance, this should be postponed until open globe is ruled out.
5. pH testing—Likely only indicated with history of chemical exposures. Most commonly tested with pH paper, urine dipsticks can also be used for testing if pH paper unavailable. Both eyes should always be tested for comparison.
6. Fluorescein exam—Fluorescein exam is essential to evaluate for corneal involvement and to evaluate for open globe (Seidel's sign).
7. Slit lamp exam—Is not indicated in all patients; however, most patients with concerns for corneal infections or defects, hypopyon, hyphema, iritis, etc. should have a slit lamp exam performed. An adequate slit lamp exam requires experience with the device. Many findings (such as cell and flare) can be subtle and are essential for accurate diagnosis.

Labs/Imaging

Labs and imaging are rarely required in the emergency department for evaluation of the red eye. Imaging may be indicated if there is a history of significant trauma and open globe or intraocular foreign body is suggested (see Ocular Imaging chapter for further information). Gram stain of conjunctival discharge may be useful, especially in the neonate and in cases of suspected gonococcal conjunctivitis. Corneal scrapings and culture are often indicated in the evaluation of keratitis; however, these are usually obtained by the ophthalmologist.

Clinical Presentations and Management of Specific Conditions (Table 6.1)

Conjunctivitis

Conjunctivitis (colloquially called "pink eye") is likely the most common cause of a red eye presenting to the emergency department. It is estimated that acute conjunctivitis affects six million people in the United States annually [1]. The majority of these conditions are benign and self-limited.

The conjunctiva is the mucous membrane that lines the interior surface of the lids and covers the sclera ending at the limbus (see Chap. 1 for further detail). Conjunctivitis universally presents with irritation and injection of this lining, causing a red appearance to the sclera. Upon closer inspection of the sclera, this red discoloration is caused by dilated blood vessels. The redness in conjunctivitis tends to concentrated peripherally, with perilimbic sparing evident (Fig. 6.1). Conjunctivitis can be bilateral or unilateral and is usually associated with increased discharge from the eye. Characterization of this discharge can help distinguish between causes. Conjunctivitis has numerous causes; these can be broadly categorized as infectious or noninfectious. Infectious causes can be further divided into viral and bacterial causes. Noninfectious conjunctivitis is predominately caused by allergic and autoimmune causes.

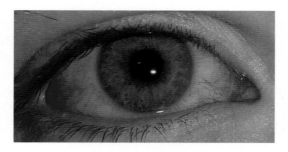

FIGURE 6.1 Conjunctivitis, note relative limbal sparing

Infectious Conjunctivitis

Infectious conjunctivitis is caused by both viral and bacterial pathogens. The incidence of each varies by age group and can be broadly separated into neonates, children, and adults.

Neonates

Neonates are at risk for bacterial conjunctival infections spreading from the mother during childbirth. These infections have the potential to causes scarring and permanent damage to the child's vision. The incidence of these infections has decreased dramatically in the developed world since introduction of routine prophylaxis at childbirth. Unfortunately, scarring from neonatal conjunctivitis (termed ophthalmia neonatorum) remains a leading cause of childhood blindness in developing countries. In the United States, topical erythromycin is the most commonly used prophylactic agent and is quite effective at preventing most maternally transmitted bacterial infections [2]. The emergency physician may still see cases of neonatal conjunctivitis in children with no perinatal care, those who refused prophylaxis, or in cases of prophylaxis failure. A gram stain should be obtained in all neonates presenting with conjunctivitis [3]. Time of onset of symptoms can be used to help identify likely causes.

Chemical Irritant Conjunctivitis

Conjunctivitis presenting in the first 2 days of life is typically chemical irritant conjunctivitis from ocular chemoprophylaxis. Gram stain can be obtained which shows white blood cells without bacterial organisms. Treatment is conservative, as symptoms will resolve spontaneously in 1–2 days [2, 3].

Gonococcal Conjunctivitis

Gonococcal conjunctivitis typically presents between 3 and 5 days after birth. Gonococcal conjunctivitis is caused by

Neisseria gonorrhoeae and is an aggressive infection that can penetrate the cornea and cause ulceration resulting in permanent loss of vision. Physical exam shows profuse purulent discharge, severe conjunctival injection, chemosis, and eyelid edema [2]. Any infant with concerns for gonococcal conjunctivitis should be treated with parenteral cefotaxime (50 mg/kg IV once) immediately [3]. Ceftriaxone should be avoided due to risk of displacement of bilirubin from albumin and precipitation of kernicterus. Conjunctival gram stain and cultures should be obtained including plating on Thayer-Martin medium and PCR if available. The emergency physician should be suspicious of systemic infection in any febrile or ill-appearing infant. All infants with concern for systemic involvement should receive lumbar puncture and full sepsis evaluation. Those with systemic signs and symptoms should be treated with a longer course of cefotaxime than isolated conjunctivitis (50 mg/kg IV Q8hrs). All infants with gonococcal conjunctivitis should be admitted and ophthalmology consulted [2, 3]. In cases of gonococcal conjunctivitis, the mother should also be treated given likely source of infection.

Chlamydial Conjunctivitis

Chlamydia trachomatis is the causative agent of neonatal chlamydial conjunctivitis. This bacterium requires a longer incubation period and does not present until 5–14 days after birth. The patient will likely have conjunctival injection and mucopurulent discharge, although typically less dramatic than those with gonococcal conjunctivitis. *Chlamydia trachomatis* is an intracellular infection and will not show up on gram stain. Historically, specialized cultures were needed to demonstrate chlamydial infection. Recent development of PCR for *Chlamydia* has shown superior sensitivity and specificity for the diagnosis as well as increased ease and speed of testing. All infants with chlamydial conjunctivitis should be treated with oral erythromycin (50 mg/kg/day divided QID). Infants should also be assessed for systemic disease stemming from chlamydial infection including pneumonia and otitis media. Neonates with isolated conjunctivitis can be discharged home with 24-h follow-up. As with gonococcal conjunctivitis, the mother should be treated empirically for chlamydia given likely source of infection [2, 3].

Other Causes of Neonatal Conjunctivitis

Bacterial conjunctivitis in neonates can be less commonly caused by nasopharyngeal organisms such as *Staphylococcus aureus*, *Streptococcus pneumoniae*, *Streptococcus viridans*, *Enterococcus* spp., and *Haemophilus* spp. These organisms can usually be found on gram stain from the conjunctiva. These organisms typically cause less severe infections and will typically resolve spontaneously. However, patients should be treated with topical antibiotics. The exception to this is infection with nontypeable *H. influenzae*. Neonates infected with this organism should receive a full septic workup, parenteral antibiotics, and admission [3]. Herpes simplex virus can also cause conjunctivitis as well as keratitis in the neonate, though it is quite rare. The diagnosis should be suspected if the neonate has any vesicular lesions anywhere on skin or mucous membranes. Dendritic lesions will be found on fluorescein exam. All patients with concern for HSV conjunctivitis should be started on parenteral acyclovir, have a lumbar puncture and full sepsis work up, and be admitted to the hospital [2, 3].

Children and Adults

Acute conjunctivitis is very common among children and adults, with greater than six million cases in the United States annually [1]. The majority of acute conjunctivitis in children is caused by bacteria (50–75% in many reports). This is in contrast to adults cases, in which viral causes are significantly more common [1, 4, 5]. Nontypeable *Haemophilus influenzae* is the most common bacterial organism isolated, followed by

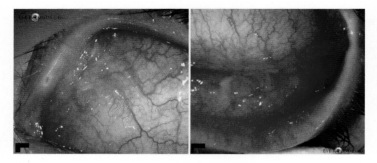

FIGURE 6.2 Classic follicular reaction of chlamydial conjunctivitis. http://webeye.ophth.uiowa.edu/eyeforum/atlas/pages/Chlamydia-trachomatis-infection.htm. The author(s)/editor(s) and publishers acknowledge the University of Iowa and EyeRounds.org for permission to reproduce this copyrighted material

Streptococcus pneumoniae and *Moraxella catarrhalis. Neisseria gonorrhoeae* and *Chlamydia trachomatis* (see Fig. 6.2) can also cause infection in sexually active adolescents and adults. *Neisseria gonorrhoeae* causes a severe hyperacute bacterial conjunctivitis. Patients with this infection may have coincident urethritis. Hyperacute bacterial conjunctivitis is characterized by copious purulent discharge, ocular pain, and visual changes. The infection can quickly lead to corneal involvement and perforation. Patients with gonococcal conjunctivitis require admission and parenteral ceftriaxone.

Adenovirus is the causative organism in 65–90% of viral conjunctivitis [1]. Herpes viruses (varicella, HSV1 and 2) are also capable of causing conjunctivitis with corneal involvement (keratitis). These will be discussed further in the keratitis section. All contact wearers with conjunctivitis should be counseled to not wear contacts until the infection completely resolves. Contact lens wearers are at increased risk of keratitis. Continued contact wear places the patient at increased risk of corneal ulcers, perforation, and permanent vision loss.

Differentiating bacterial conjunctivitis from viral conjunctivitis can be difficult. Symptoms and physical exam cannot reliably distinguish these diseases [6]. Testing such as gram stain, culture, and PCR are time-consuming, poorly sensitive, and not indicated in the vast majority of conjunctivitis. This quandary has led many physicians to treat all cases of conjunctivitis with topical antibiotics. Unfortunately, when studied this approach has been shown to have no benefit [4]. It has, however, caused a predictable increase in resistance patterns among causative bacterial [4, 5]. This is likely due to the fact that the majority of bacterial conjunctivitis resolves spontaneously without complications. Additionally, studies have shown minimal benefit to treating culture-proven bacterial conjunctivitis with topical antibiotics [4, 7]. Therefore, treating all cases of conjunctivitis with antibiotics (the majority of which will be viral) is not likely to have benefit. A "watch and wait" approach may be reasonable in most uncomplicated conjunctivitis [8]. However, antibiotics should be started in all patients with severe symptoms, contact lens wearers, and patients with concerns for gonococcal or chlamydial infection [1].

If the decision to start topical antibiotics is made there is no clear superiority of one agent over another in the general population. Reasonable choices include erythromycin, trimethoprim-polymyxin B, or bacitracin [1, 8]. Fluoroquinolones should be avoided as first line to avoid creating resistance. The exception to this is contact lens wearers who should have a fluoroquinolone started given the high incidence of *Pseudomonas* infection [8].

Noninfectious Conjunctivitis

Allergic Conjunctivitis

Allergic conjunctivitis is exceptionally common; some estimates assert that 40% of the US population suffers from allergic conjunctivitis [1]. The majority of these cases are mild, and most patients do not seek medical attention. Patients with allergic conjunctivitis will often have a history of atopy. Patients describe bilateral itching eye itching and tearing as the predominant symptoms. Physical exam shows relatively mild injection, thin mucoid discharge, and chemosis. Other symptoms of seasonal allergies may be present—rhinorrhea, sneezing, etc. The diagnosis is clinical, and treatment includes topical antihistamines and primary care follow-up for further management [3].

Autoimmune Conjunctivitis

The majority of rheumatologic diseases can present with ocular manifestations, most commonly uveitis, scleritis, or episcleritis. Autoimmune causes of isolated conjunctivitis are relatively rare. Kawasaki's disease (KD) is an important cause of autoimmune conjunctivitis in the pediatric population. KD is a medium vessel vasculitis which presents predominantly in children under the age of 8 years old, with 85% of cases presenting under the age of 5 [9]. Bilateral conjunctivitis is present in greater than 90% of cases of KD [10]. Typical KD is diagnosed with clinical criteria. Patients must have fever for greater than 5 days and four out of five of the following symptoms:

- Bilateral conjunctival injection
- Mucous membrane involvement including: strawberry tongue, erythematous, cracked lips, oropharyngeal erythema
- Polymorphous rash
- Extremity involvement including: edema of hands and feet, periungual desquamation
- Cervical adenopathy

Atypical KD also exists in which patients do not meet all criteria. Therefore, providers should maintain high degree of suspicion for KD despite not meeting all criteria. KD is a self-limited disease; however, patients are at high risk for serious complications including coronary aneurysms [9]. Inflammatory markers should be obtained in all patients in whom KD is suspected. All patients with KD require admission, oral aspirin, intravenous immunoglobulin (IVIG), and cardiology consultation for echocardiography [3, 9].

Reactive arthritis (previously called Reiter's syndrome) is a rare postinfectious complication of some enteral infections (typically *Salmonella*, *Shigella*, *Campylobacter*, or *Yersinia*) or genitourinary infections (typically *Chlamydia*). Symptoms usually present after initial infection has resolved and can include mono- or polyarticular arthritis, dactylitis, mucocutaneous lesions, and ocular manifestations including conjunctivitis, among other symptoms [11]. In a series of 186 patients with reactive arthritis, ocular involvement was found in 20% of patients [12]. Diagnosis is made clinically based on recent infection and distribution of postinfectious symptoms. Treatment is mainly symptomatic and may include NSAIDs for arthritis. Treatment of underlying infection should be considered if not completely resolved; however, a 2013 meta-analysis found no clear benefit to antibiotics in the resolution of reactive arthritis [13]. There is no clear treatment for ocular involvement. Patients with reactive arthritis should be referred to a rheumatologist for further management. Those with chronic symptoms may require immunosuppressive agents for control of symptoms [11].

Keratitis

Keratitis refers to inflammation of the layers of the cornea. Patients may present with both conjunctivitis and keratitis; therefore, it is imperative to complete a full ocular exam and rule out keratitis before a sole diagnosis of conjunctivitis is made. Keratitis has both infectious and noninfectious causes. The CDC estimates there are approximately one million clinic and emergency department visits annually for keratitis in the United States, leading to $175 million dollars in direct healthcare expenditure on the disease [14]. The single most important risk factor for keratitis is contact lens wear. Patients with keratitis will present with redness, eye pain, photophobia, foreign body sensation, and possibly blurred vision if lesions are in the visual axis or there is associated iritis [15]. History should focus on timing of symptoms, contact lens use, occupational and exposure history, and any history of trauma to the eye. Diagnosis will be made with fluorescein and slit lamp exam showing characteristic fluorescein staining. By integrating history, physical, and exam, the emergency clinician should be able to categorize the type of keratitis present. All patients with concern for infectious keratitis should urgently see an ophthalmologist given potential for severe corneal scarring and vision loss.

Infectious Keratitis

Bacterial Keratitis

Bacterial keratitis is a medical emergency. Patients usually have at least one risk factor for the disease. The predominant risk factor for bacterial keratitis is contact lens wear; poor hygiene and infrequent lens changing increase the risk. Other risk factors include corneal trauma or surgery, immunosuppression, cocaine use, and topical corticosteroids. Bacterial keratitis can form in those without risk factors, usually from particularly virulent organisms such as *Neisseria*, *Diphtheria*, and *Listeria* species [16]. Patients will present with symptoms of keratitis (redness, pain, photophobia, etc.). Slit lamp and fluorescein findings are heterogeneous and include a corneal infiltrate; a focal hazy or cloudy appearance to the cornea, corneal ulcer with fluorescein uptake (Figs. 6.3 and 6.4), multifocal keratopathy, and, in severe cases, a hypopyon may be visible. All patients with suspected bacterial keratitis should have emergent ophthalmologic consultation for scrapings and culture of infection [15]. If ophthalmology is not readily available, broad-spectrum topical antibiotics should be started; options include a fluoroquinolone (ofloxacin, moxifloxacin, or

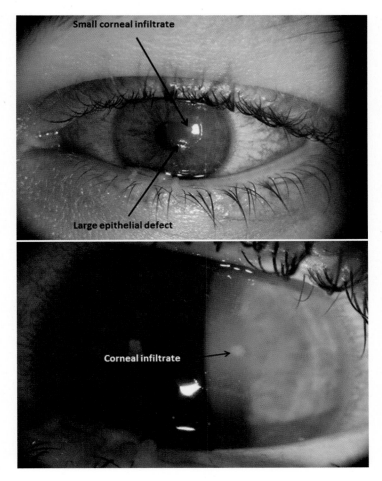

FIGURE 6.3 Bacterial keratitis—note hazy corneal infiltrate

ciprofloxacin) or combination therapy with cephalosporin and aminoglycoside [15, 16]. Approximately 95% of infections will respond to appropriately chosen initial antibiotics; therefore, culture results are often unnecessary [16].

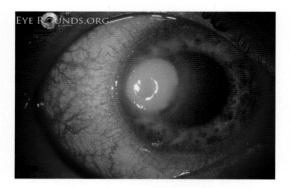

FIGURE 6.4 Large corneal infiltrate and ulcer due to *Pseudomonas.*
http://webeye.ophth.uiowa.edu/eyeforum/atlas/pages/pseudomo-
nas-keratitis-34.html. The author(s)/editor(s) and publishers
acknowledge the University of Iowa and EyeRounds.org for permission to reproduce this copyrighted material

Viral Keratitis

Herpes Simplex Keratoconjunctivitis

Herpes simplex virus 1 and 2 (HSV1 and 2) are exceptionally
common viruses worldwide. In many parts of the world,
nearly every person is infected with HSV1 by adulthood.
These viruses cause a primary outbreak syndrome which may
include fever, malaise, orolabial or genital vesicles, and potentially ocular involvement. After the primary infection sub-
sides, the virus remains dormant in nerve ganglion and
reactivates with certain triggers. These can include fever,
menses, sunlight, and emotional stress. Reactivation occurs in
27% of people at 1 year and 60% at 20 years post infection.
Recurrences typically produce a less severe illness than the
primary outbreak [17].

Ocular manifestations differ in primary outbreak and
recurrences as well. Primary HSV is typically associated with
blepharoconjunctivitis, often confused with adenovirus infection. Keratitis in the primary outbreak is rare but may occur

3–5% of the time. These symptoms heal without scarring or permanent damage. Immunocompromised patients may suffer more severe disease and bilateral symptoms. HSV recurrences can be associated with infection of all parts of the eye but is commonly associated with keratitis. Globally, there are approximately one million cases of herpetic keratitis per year [18]. The classic finding on fluorescein exam is a branching dendritic pattern with terminal bulbs (Fig. 6.5). Other patterns can be observed in severe cases including a geographic ulcer—a large corneal ulcer-like defect, usually with dendritic pattern at the periphery (Fig. 6.6). Geographic ulcers are typically associated with topical steroid use or immunosuppression. These lesions often heal with scarring, leading to permanent visual damage [17, 18]. Diagnosis is typically made clinically; however, if the diagnosis is in doubt, viral cultures can be obtained.

Treatment for vesicular skin lesions is oral antivirals (acyclovir, valacyclovir, etc.). Patients with HSV keratitis should be treated with either oral acyclovir or topical antivirals

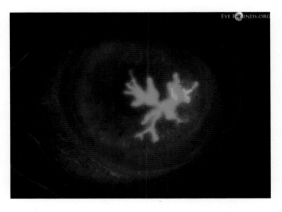

Figure 6.5 Dendritic lesion due to HSV keratitis. http://webeye. ophth.uiowa.edu/eyeforum/atlas/pages/HSV-keratitis/HSV-fluor-LRG.jpg. The author(s)/editor(s) and publishers acknowledge the University of Iowa and EyeRounds.org for permission to reproduce this copyrighted material

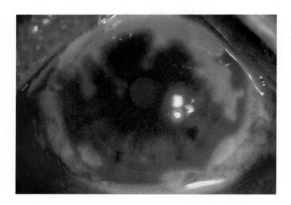

FIGURE 6.6 Geographic ulcer. By Hee K Yang, Young K Han, Won R Wee, Jin H Lee and Ji W Kwon; Department of Ophthalmology, Seoul National University College of Medicine, Seoul, Korea— License: http://www.jmedicalcasereports.com/content/5/1/328 Image: http://www.jmedicalcasereports.com/content/5/1/328/figure/F1, CC BY 2.5, https://commons.wikimedia.org/w/index.php?curid=20977438

(trifluridine, acyclovir ganciclovir, or brivudine). A 2015 Cochrane review found no difference between any topical agents or oral acyclovir in the treatment of herpetic keratitis [18]. Many patients prefer treatment with oral acyclovir given ease of dosing. Studies demonstrate no benefit of addition of oral acyclovir to trifluridine alone; therefore, treatment with oral or topical antiviral medications alone is appropriate [19, 20]. Topical corticosteroids have also shown faster resolution of lesions; however, application of topical steroids increases risk of secondary bacterial and other complications. Studies have shown no adverse effects from delaying corticosteroids [17]. It may be prudent for the emergency physician to refer corticosteroid use to the ophthalmologist. Erythromycin ointment may be prescribed to prevent secondary bacterial infection. All patients presenting with HSV keratitis need follow-up with an ophthalmologist within 24–48 h [15].

Herpes Zoster Ophthalmicus

Herpes zoster ophthalmicus is a complication of reactivation of the herpes zoster virus which is the causative agent in chickenpox and shingles. Infection usually occurs during childhood; the patient has the chickenpox syndrome and is asymptomatic for many years. The virus is stored in nerve ganglion and can reactivate later in life causing the shingles syndrome [15]. Childhood vaccination for chickenpox and shingles vaccine for older adults has decreased incidence of the disease [21]. Unfortunately, shingles remains common in the older population with approximately one in the three individuals being affected in their lifetime. Herpes zoster ophthalmicus refers to reactivation of the virus in the trigeminal V1 distribution. This can lead to involvement of the tip of the nose (called Hutchinson's sign) and ipsilateral ocular involvement. Zoster ophthalmicus occurs in 10–20% of reactivations and is more common in immune suppressed patients [21]. Patients may complain of fever, malaise, burning sensation preceding rash, blurred vision, and photophobia. A facial rash may be evident on the tip of the nose and eyelid or, more rarely, over the cheek and mandible if the V2 or V3 branches are involved [15] (Fig. 6.7). Ocular involvement is heterogeneous; keratitis may be evident on fluorescein staining, classically demonstrating a branching pseudodendritic pattern-branching without terminal bulb formation (Fig. 6.8). The patient may also have ocular involvement without keratitis including uveitis, choroiditis, and retinitis. Treatment includes oral antiviral medications (acyclovir, famciclovir, or valacyclovir) [15, 21]. Routine administration of oral glucocorticoids is no longer recommended given recent meta-analysis showing no effect on quality of life or postherpetic neuralgia [22]. Topical steroids may improve ophthalmologic involvement; however, these should not be given without consultation from an ophthalmologist given high rates of complications with topical steroids. Erythromycin ointment is recommended in all patients with corneal involvement to

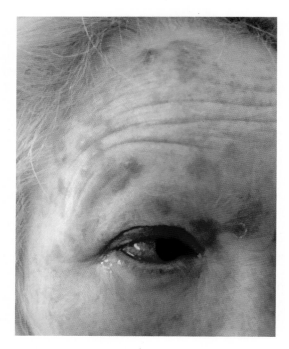

FIGURE 6.7 Herpes Zoster ophthalmicus. Note skin lesions and ocular involvement. Photo credit: By Burntfingers—Own work, CC BY-SA 4.0, https://commons.wikimedia.org/w/index.php?curid=38576178

lubricate the eye and prevent secondary bacterial infection [15, 21]. Consider IV antivirals and admission for all patients with immunosuppression, systemic illness, optic nerve, or cranial nerve involvement. Patients with retinal or optic nerve involvement warrant urgent consultation with ophthalmologists [21]. Patients discharged home should have close follow-up with an ophthalmologist.

Epidemic Keratoconjunctivitis

Epidemic keratoconjunctivitis (EKC) is a syndrome produced by several strands of adenovirus. The virus is extremely contagious and tends to occur in epidemics [15, 23].

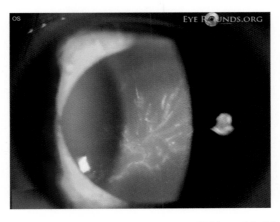

FIGURE 6.8 Pseudodendritic lesion due to VZV keratitis. Note lack of terminal bulbs on branches. http://webeye.ophth.uiowa.edu/eye-forum/atlas/pages/VZV-keratitis/VZV-keratitis-LRG.jpg. The author(s)/editor(s) and publishers acknowledge the University of Iowa and EyeRounds.org for permission to reproduce this copyrighted material

In 2008–2010, there were multiple outbreaks in the United States totaling 411 cases. The majority of cases were health-care associated, usually associated with transmission via ophthalmologic equipment during examination [23]. The virus is resistant to 70% isopropyl alcohol, and disposable gloves and equipment should be used in an outbreak whenever possible. Care should be taken to properly sterilize all non-disposable equipment used to examine patients during an outbreak. EKC is often preceded by a prodrome of fever, myalgias, cough, and malaise [15]. Ocular involvement begins as severe conjunctivitis, similar to other adenovirus infections. Several days after the onset of conjunctivitis the patient develops keratitis [23, 24]. This is usually appears on fluorescein exam as diffuse punctate keratitis [15, 24] (Fig. 6.9). EKC is a self-limited disease with symptoms usually lasting 7–21 days followed by complete resolution. Treatment is supportive [23]. Unfortunately, some patients may develop subendothelial infiltrates that persist from months to years and cause some degree of visual impairment [24]. Patients with severe or

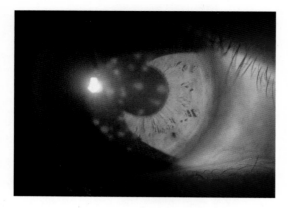

Figure 6.9 Punctate keratitis associated with adenovirus (Imrankabirhossain — Own work, CC BY-SA 4.0, https://commons. wikimedia.org/w/index.php?curid=59071923)

prolonged symptoms or significant visual changes should have follow-up with an ophthalmologist.

Parasitic Keratitis

Worldwide parasitic keratitis is a common and devastating disease. Onchocerciasis (also known as river blindness) is the second leading cause of blindness worldwide, infecting more than 37 million people and rendering at least 500,000 blind. In the developed world, parasitic keratitis is a rare disease. This review will focus on parasitic keratitis in the developed world. *Acanthamoeba* keratitis (AK) is the only significant cause of parasitic keratitis in the United States with an estimated incidence of 0.15 cases per million in the United States [25] (Fig. 6.10). Contact lens use is the primary risk factor with 85–88% of cases presenting in contact lens wearers. Soft contact lens and poor hygiene are additional risk factors. AK accounts for less than 5% of infectious keratitis in contact lens wearers, reflecting the much higher incidence of bacterial or viral causes. AK can occur in noncontact lens wearers, usually associated with trauma and soil contamination of the eye, such

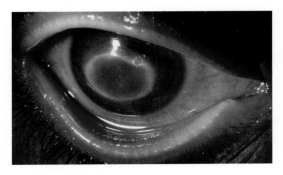

FIGURE 6.10 Classic ring infiltrate due to *Acanthamoeba* keratitis. http://webeye.ophth.uiowa.edu/eyeforum/atlas/pages/acanthamoeba/acanthamoeba-LRG.jpg. The author(s)/editor(s) and publishers acknowledge the University of Iowa and EyeRounds.org for permission to reproduce this copyrighted material

as in agricultural workers [25]. Prompt diagnosis of this disease is imperative. Delayed diagnosis leads to irreversible damage and permanent vision damage or loss. Severe pain, out of proportion to exam, is common in AK (however, pain-free cases have been reported) [25, 26]. The diagnosis is difficult to make, and the disease is often misdiagnosed for an extended period of time [27]. Definitive diagnosis is likely not possible in the emergency department, as culture and specialized scrapings and stains are required [25, 26]. This reflects the importance of follow-up with an ophthalmologist in all cases of infective keratitis in contact lens wearers. Emergency physicians should be familiar with the risk factors for this disease and relay concerns to the consulting physician. The diagnosis should also be considered in patients presenting to the emergency department with previously diagnosed bacterial or viral keratitis who have worsening pain or symptoms despite treatment. While exceptionally rare, the diagnosis should also be considered in noncontact lens wearers presenting with severe keratitis and risk factors mentioned above. Treatment is challenging, and successful treatment decreases with delayed diagnosis. Treatment should be deferred to the ophthalmologist, as the diagnosis will not be made in the emergency department.

Fungal Keratitis

Fungal keratitis is a common disease worldwide and predominates in tropical regions of the globe. In the United States, the disease is relatively rare; however, the incidence varies widely based on region of the United States. Fungal organisms are found to be the cause of 6–20% of infectious keratitis in the United States with highest incidence in tropical regions [28]. Rates as high as 35% of infectious keratitis have been reported in South Florida [29]. Risk factors for fungal keratitis include trauma—particularly trauma with vegetative material (tree branches, etc.), soft contact lens use, topical corticosteroid use, and immunosuppression [28, 30, 31]. Patients present with symptoms similar to all other causes of keratitis—pain, photophobia, foreign body sensation, and blurred vision. Slit lamp and fluorescein exam shows a corneal infiltrate and often an ulcer. Slit lamp findings are heterogeneous depending on the organism involved and extent of infection [30]. Fungal keratitis may demonstrate a feathery edge to the ulcer [32] (Fig. 6.11). Diagnosis will not be made in the emergency department as this requires specialized scrapings and cultures. Treatment options are limited, and medical treatment fails in approx. 15–20% of cases [30, 31]. Surgical intervention is required in 15–40% of cases [28, 31]. The emergency physician will not definitely diagnose or treat this disease, but it is important to consider the disease when risk factors or physical findings consistent with the disease are present. Emergent referral to an ophthalmologist may lead to earlier diagnosis and treatment and decrease rates of medical failure.

Noninfectious Keratitis

Ultraviolet (UV) Keratitis

Corneal epithelial cells are, as all other epithelial cells, susceptible to damage from UV radiation. Significant UV radiation exposure can cause corneal cell death and diffuse keratitis.

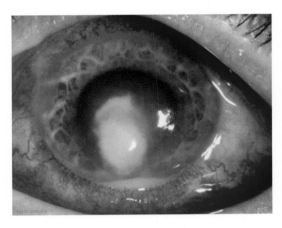

FIGURE 6.11 Fungal keratitis—note feathery appearance to edge of infiltrate. Also note small hypopyon. http://webeye.ophth.uiowa. edu/eyeforum/atlas/pages/Fungal-keratitis/fungal-keratitis-201208-LRG.jpg. The author(s)/editor(s) and publishers acknowledge the University of Iowa and EyeRounds.org for permission to reproduce this copyrighted material

Risk factors include occupational or recreational activities that involve significant UV exposure. Welding without proper eye protection is the typical occupational exposure (called arc eye). Recreational exposures include high-altitude snow sports such as glacial travel (called snow blindness) and exposure in tanning beds [15, 33]. Several unusual epidemics have been observed in the United States (as recently as 2013) after improper lighting that emit high levels of UV radiation was installed in several school gymnasiums. In one episode, 242 patients developed UV keratitis from a broken metal halide bulb [34]. The emergency physician has an important role in the recognition of outbreaks and can assist in identifying causes.

UV keratitis presents with significant pain, photophobia, and foreign body sensation, similar to other forms of keratitis. Symptoms are typically bilateral, usually present 6–12 h after initial exposure [15]. Examination shows corneal edema, conjunctival injection, and tearing. Fluorescein exam

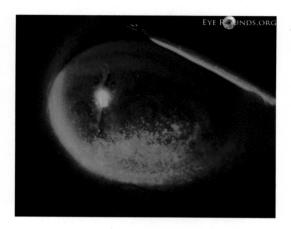

FIGURE 6.12 Diffuse fluorescein uptake due to punctate keratitis related to UV exposure. http://webeye.ophth.uiowa.edu/eyeforum/ atlas/pages/punctate-epithelial-erosions/Exposure-PEE-LRG.jpg. The author(s)/editor(s) and publishers acknowledge the University of Iowa and EyeRounds.org for permission to reproduce this copyrighted material

shows diffuse punctate keratopathy [15, 33] (Fig. 6.12). Treatment is supportive and may include cycloplegics and oral analgesia. Erythromycin ointment may be given to prevent secondary bacterial infection [15]. UV keratitis is self-limited, and complete healing is typically observed with 36 h. Scarring and visual impairment is rare [15, 33].

Corneal Abrasion

Corneal abrasions are a common diagnosis, accounting for approximately 10% of eye-related visits in the emergency department [35]. The cornea is richly innervated, and abrasions are extremely painful [15]. Corneal abrasions are generally minor injuries; however, thorough evaluation must be performed to rule out concerning diagnoses such as open globe, intraocular or corneal foreign body, or hyphema.

Evaluation should include a thorough history including a description of trauma, history of contact lens use, vision changes, etc. Abrasions are often caused by minor trauma (fingernails, tree branches, etc.); patients usually recall the trauma as pain present nearly instantaneously after injury. Symptoms include pain, a foreign body sensation, blurred vision, and photophobia if iritis is present. Particular attention should be paid to mechanisms that may lead to retained foreign body (grinding, hammering, etc.) or penetrating trauma. Pain should be treated with topical anesthetics such as tetracaine (0.5%) or proparacaine (0.5%) prior to examination.

Examination should include visual acuity, fluorescein staining, and slit lamp exam. Eyelids should also be everted to evaluate for foreign body retained under lid. Fluorescein exam will demonstrate uptake at site of corneal abrasion (Fig. 6.13). Fluorescein exam can also be used to evaluate for evidence of open globe. Seidel's sign (fluorescein flowing down eye from site of penetration) may be present in cases of open globe. The slit lamp exam can be used to locate and measure corneal abrasions and evaluate for corneal foreign body,

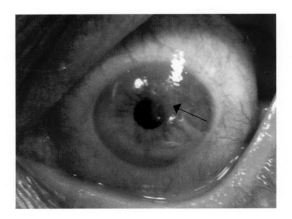

Figure 6.13 Corneal abrasion with fluorescein uptake. Photo credit: By James Heilman, MD—Own work, CC BY-SA 3.0, https://commons.wikimedia.org/w/index.php?curid=11918476

rust ring, etc. The clinician should note the location of the abrasion on the cornea, as those in the visual axis are more concerning than those located peripherally.

Management of uncomplicated corneal abrasions includes pain control and prevention of secondary infection. Topical NSAIDs (diclofenac, ketorolac, indomethacin, etc.) have been shown to be effective for pain control and safe in the setting of corneal abrasion [36]. Topical anesthetics are extremely effective at controlling pain from corneal abrasions. Unfortunately, serious risks from repeated application of these drugs exist. Topical anesthetics have been shown to be toxic to the corneal epithelium, and routine use can predispose to serious infection. Serious morbidity including vision loss has occurred due to topical anesthetic overuse. Recently, several trials have evaluated the safety of using topical anesthetics (0.05% proparacaine, 1% tetracaine) in patients presenting to the emergency department with corneal abrasions. These trials have shown relative safety of this method with variable improvement of pain scores [35, 37, 38]. The use of topical anesthetics is still controversial, and most textbooks recommend against their use [15, 35]. If topical anesthetic is used, close follow-up should be arranged to ensure adequate healing. Oral analgesics may also be considered (acetaminophen, ibuprofen, etc.). Topical antibiotics are often prescribed. A large trial performed in Nepal showed decreased rates of secondary bacterial infection with routine use of topical antibiotics [39].

Historically, cycloplegics and eye patches were applied to the affected eye in all cases of corneal abrasion. Recent studies, including a Cochrane review of 12 studies, showed no improvement in pain with patching [40]. Patching may also increase the risk of secondary infection and is therefore no longer routinely recommended [41]. Few studies have evaluated the effect of cycloplegics for corneal abrasions. A 1996 showed no difference in pain control between the application of homatropine (cycloplegic) and lubricant eye drops (polyvinyl alcohol) [42]. Cycloplegics may be considered for large abrasions or those with concomitant iritis; however, routine use is not recommended [15, 41].

Uncomplicated corneal abrasions typically heal completely within 72 h [15, 41]. Scarring may occur with deep corneal abrasions, though this is rare [41]. Patients with large abrasions (>2 mm) or abrasions in the central visual axis should be referred to ophthalmologist for recheck of wound in 24 h [15]. Patients who wear contact lens should be counseled to avoid contact lens use until symptoms completely resolve.

Subconjunctival Hemorrhage

Subconjunctival hemorrhage (SCH) is a common benign condition. Blood vessels of the conjunctival are fragile and easily ruptured by minor trauma, increased venous pressure (from sneezing, coughing, vomiting, etc.), or inflammation [15, 43, 44]. Clinically this condition appears as a flat, sharply demarcated collection of blood present in the conjunctiva (Fig. 6.14). Risk factors include contact lens wear, anticoagulation, hypertension, and systemic vascular diseases [43, 44]. This is a painless condition; thus, patients with pain should be investigated for other causes such as corneal abrasion, open globe, or traumatic iritis. All patients with pain or history of trauma should have fluorescein exam to evaluate for corneal abrasion or

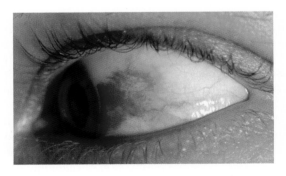

FIGURE 6.14 Subconjunctival hemorrhage. Photo credit: Daniel Flather—Own work, CC BY-SA 3.0. https://commons.wikimedia.org/w/index.php?curid=15651313

open globe. Consider coagulation studies for patients on anti-coagulation presenting with spontaneous or persistent SCH. Isolated SCH requires no treatment, only reassurance. SCH should spontaneously resolve within 2 weeks [15].

Steven-Johnson Syndrome and Toxic Epidermal Necrolysis

Steven-Johnson syndrome (SJS) and toxic epidermal necrolysis (TEN) represent a spectrum of immune-mediated dermatologic disease. These conditions lead to large-scale keratinocyte death and epidermal sloughing including skin and mucous membrane surfaces (oral, vaginal, gastrointestinal, respiratory, etc.). The diseases is called SJS when <10% of body surface area (BSA) is involved; TEN is defined as >30% BSA. Disease falling between this 10–30% BSA involvement is referred to as SJS/TENS overlap syndrome. These diseases are rare (incidence 0.6–6 cases per million) but lead to high rates of morbidity and mortality [45, 46]. Mortality rates for the SJS-TENS spectrum are high, with rates from 1% to 5% in SJS to 25–50% in TEN [46]. These diseases are most often caused by an idiosyncratic reaction to medications. Over 200 medications have been implicated, most often sulfonamide antibiotics, aromatic antiepileptics (phenytoin, carbamazepine, etc.), beta-lactam antibiotics, and NSAIDs. Rarely, SJS/TENs may have infectious causes such as herpes or *Mycoplasma* infections, although this is controversial [46].

Ocular involvement is common in the SJS/TENS spectrum with reported rates from 50 to 88% [47]. Ocular symptoms may include conjunctivitis, cornea ulceration, and complete sloughing of epithelium of eye and eyelid (Fig. 6.15). Severe scarring is common, and long-term visual impairment occurs in up to one third of survivors of the disease [47]. The mainstay of treatment for this disease is discontinuation of offending agent and supportive care. Treatment for ocular involvement is controversial and may include topic steroids, IVIG, or other immunosuppresants [45–47]. These diseases should not be managed by an emergency physician. All patients with SJS/TENS should be admitted to a burn unit. The emergency physician should evaluate

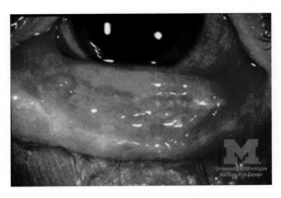

FIGURE 6.15 SJS associated conjunctivitis. Photo credit: By Jonathan Trobe, M.D., University of Michigan Kellogg Eye Center http://www.kellogg.umich.edu/theeyeshaveit/acquired/conjunctivitis.html,   CC BY 3.0, https://commons.wikimedia.org/w/index.php?curid=8406623

for ocular involvement with fluorescein staining. All patients with ocular involvement should have an urgent ophthalmologic consultation, with the goal of reducing long-term sequelae.

Iritis

The uveal tract (middle layer of the eye) can be divided into anterior and posterior sections. The anterior section is made up of the iris and the ciliary body. Anterior uveitis refers to inflammation of either of these components; this can also be called iritis (when only the iris is inflamed) or iridocyclitis (inflammation of both iris and ciliary body). Iritis is the most common term used in the emergency department. The incidence of uveitis is 25–341/100,000 depending on the population [48–51]. Anterior uveitis is by far the most common, making up 92% of cases of uveitis. Despite its relative rarity, uveitis is estimate to cause 10–15% of total cases of blindness in the United States [52] or as many as 30,000 cases per year [50]. Iritis, while painful and debilitating, is not a true medical emergency, but does need follow-up with an ophthalmologist [15]. Morbidity from this disease is caused by the chronic and recurrent nature of inflammation.

The differential for iritis is quite broad. Iritis often occurs with ocular infections, systemic autoimmune diseases, and after ocular trauma. It is commonly seen in a variety of ocular infections including keratitis (any cause, most commonly herpetic infections), CMV retinitis, etc. It may complicate systemic viral or bacterial infections with common pathogens such as Epstein-Barr virus, influenza, and syphilis, as well as rare diseases such as cat-scratch fever, brucellosis, and West Nile virus [51, 53]. Iritis is commonly caused by postinfectious immune-mediated inflammation, most commonly after streptococcal infections. Systemic autoimmune diseases account for the majority of iritis with a diagnosed cause (non-idiopathic). Iritis is associated with a wide variety of autoimmune disease including inflammatory bowel disease, ankylosing spondylitis, juvenile arthritis, and Behcet's syndrome [51]. Iritis can occur after ocular surgery and with other forms of ocular trauma.

History should focus on recent infections or trauma, autoimmune history, and a thorough review of symptoms. Patients report pain, redness, blurred vision, and photophobia. Discharge is uncommon with isolated iritis, but may occur if other infectious processes are present. Examination may show conjunctival injection with the most intense inflammation at the limbus (called ciliary flush) [15, 51]. The affected pupil will often be miotic and sluggishly reactive to light (Fig. 6.16). Consensual photophobia (pain in affected eye when light shine in unaffected eye) is the classic exam finding due to consensual pupillary constriction. Fluorescein exam should be performed to evaluate for keratitis, corneal abrasions, etc. Slit lamp examina-

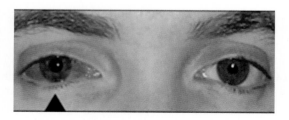

Figure 6.16 Unilateral iritis, note significant conjunctival injection and asymmetric pupil size (can see miosis or mydriasis, typically with sluggish light response). By Paul S UK—Own work, CC BY-SA 3.0, https://commons.wikimedia.org/w/index.php?curid=1660576

tion will show white blood cells suspended in the anterior chamber, referred to as cell and flare (often subtle).

Patients with iritis should be thoroughly evaluated for infectious and traumatic causes. Underlying causes (keratitis, corneal abrasion, systemic infections, etc.) should be treated and follow-up scheduled as indicated. Iritis is treated with long-acting cycloplegic medications such as homatropine to block pupillary constriction and reduce pain [15, 51]. Patients with isolated iritis with no apparent cause or clear autoimmune cause should follow up with an ophthalmologist in 24–48 h for further evaluation [15].

Chemical Burn

Ocular chemical burns are true ophthalmologic emergencies. Patients will usually present immediately after known exposure to a chemical. Symptoms include blepharospasm, redness, and severe pain. The clinician should attempt to identify the irritant; however, early irrigation is of utmost importance. Irrigation takes priority over examination and testing. Immediately after a chemical exposure is identified, irrigation should start with 1–2 liters of isotonic solution (lactated ringers, normal saline, etc.). Comparison of several isotonic solutions showed no difference in normalization of pH [54]. A topical anesthetic can be applied prior to irrigation for pain control. A Morgan lens or other device designed for ocular irrigation may be helpful; if not available, manual flushing should be initiated. Irrigation should not be delayed for visual acuity, pH testing, or physical examination. After irrigation has begun a more thorough history can be obtained focusing on timing of exposure, substance exposure, and symptoms after event [15, 55, 56].

Chemical burns are generally caused by alkali or acidic exposures. Alkali exposures cause significantly more damage as alkaline solutions cause liquefactive necrosis allowing for deep penetration into tissues and significant damage. Acidic exposures tend to be more superficial. Damage by acids causes coagulation of proteins which acts as a barrier to deep penetration [55, 56].

Irrigation should continue until pH testing shows return to physiologic pH (7.3–7.4). Testing should be performed every

30 minutes during irrigation. After irrigation has finished, a thorough examination should be completed. Patients may have chemosis, conjunctival injection, and corneal opacification. More severe injuries may demonstrate scleral whitening due to ischemia and vasospasm. Visual testing should be performed, as well as fluorescein and slit lamp exam. Fluorescein exam will show uptake in areas of corneal damage. Extent of uptake should be documented, as an ophthalmologist will follow uptake to evaluate for healing. Slit lamp exam may show cell and flare due to inflammation of the anterior chamber if penetration occurred [15, 55, 56].

All patients with significant ocular burns warrant emergent ophthalmologist consultation for further management. Patients with no uptake on fluorescein exam and no anterior chamber findings may be treated as outpatients. These patients should be treated with a topical antibiotic ointment and should follow up with an ophthalmologist in 24–48 h [15].

For a more in depth review of ocular burns, please see the chapter entitled "Ocular Burns and Exposures."

Pearls/Pitfalls

- The incidence of viral and bacterial conjunctivitis varies by age. All neonates should have gram stain and likely be treated (exception is chemical irritant conjunctivitis). In children and adults, a watch and wait strategy may be appropriate, as most cases viral and bacterial resolve spontaneously.
- In all patients with keratitis, consider rare causes such as *Acanthamoeba* and fungal keratitis. These are rare diagnosis but cause significant morbidity if missed.
- Diagnoses may coexist (IE conjunctivitis and keratitis, corneal abrasion, and subconjunctival hemorrhage). It is important to perform a thorough exam to evaluate for all dangerous pathology.
- Do not delay irrigation in chemical burns for history, exam, or testing.
- All contact lens users with ocular pathology should be instructed to avoid contact lens use until symptoms completely resolve.

TABLE 6.1 Quick reference table

Disease	General info	Symptoms	Physical findings	Testing indicated	Treatment
Conjunctivitis		Mild pain, itching, blurred vision	• Injection of conjunctiva • Discharge (watery, mucopurulent)		
Neonates					
Chemical	Present in first 2 days of life, from chemoprophylaxis		• Mild conjunctival injection	Gram stain	Supportive
Gonococcal	Presents between 3 and 5 days after birth		• Copious mucopurulent discharge • Significant chemosis • Conjunctival injection	Gram stain, culture	Intravenous cefotaxime. Also treat mother for gonorrhea

(continued)

TABLE 6.1 (continued)

Disease	General info	Symptoms	Physical findings	Testing indicated	Treatment
Chlamydial	Presents 5–14 days after birth		• Mucopurulent discharge • Conjunctival injection	Gram stain, PCR	Oral erythromycin. Treat mother for chlamydia
Children + adults					All patients must remove contact lenses until symptoms resolve
Viral	Most common cause overall. Adults > children	Ocular itching, blurred vision, matting of eyelids	• Discharge (watery, mucopurulent) • Conjunctival injection • May have URI symptoms • Difficult to distinguish from bacterial causes	None indicated	Supportive

Bacterial	Children>adults	Ocular itching, blurred vision, matting of eyelids	• Similar to viral • Exception-gonococcal Copious Discharge Chemosis Severe conjunctival injection	Only if suspicion for gonococcal. Gram stain, culture	• Gonococcal- IV ceftriaxone • Routine treatment for nongonococcal, non-chlamydial may not be required • Contact lens wearers—topical fluoroquinolone
Allergic	Very common, few seek medical care. Typically mild symptoms	Ocular itching, tearing sneezing, other symptoms of seasonal allergies	• Conjunctival injection • Thin mucoid discharge • Chemosis	None indicated	Topical antihistamines

(continued)

Table 6.1 (continued)

Disease	General info	Symptoms	Physical findings	Testing indicated	Treatment
Autoimmune	Rare. Consider Kawasaki's disease (children), reactive arthritis, etc.	Symptoms of underlying rheumatic condition such as myalgias, rashes, etc.	• Findings of underlying rheumatic condition	Testing for underlying autoimmune condition	Treat underlying condition
Keratitis	Inflammation of cornea. Contact lens wearers particularly at risk	Pain, photophobia. Blurred vision	All forms have corneal fluorescein uptake, may have hazy corneal infiltrate. Pattern may distinguish causes	Fluorescein exam, slit lamp exam	All patient must remove contact lenses until symptoms resolve
Bacterial			• Corneal ulcer often present • Hypopyon may be present in severe cases	Cultures obtained by ophthalmologist	Emergent ophthalmology consult. Broad-spectrum topical antibiotics

Viral	Many organisms possible. HSV, herpes zoster most common	May include fever and skin rash	• HSV: Dendritic lesions, geographic ulcer, oral/genital rash • Zoster: Pseudodendritic lesions, dermatomal rash, Hutchison's sign	Usually diagnosed by exam	• HSV: Oral acyclovir or topical antivirals • Zoster: Oral antivirals • Erythromycin ointment to prevent secondary infection • Topical steroids should only be given by ophthalmologist • Urgent follow-up with ophthalmologist
Fungal	Rare, more common in tropical climates		May have corneal ulcer with feathery edges	Very difficult to diagnose, requires ophthalmologist	Will be initiated by ophthalmologist

(continued)

TABLE 6.1 (continued)

Disease	General info	Symptoms	Physical findings	Testing indicated	Treatment
Parasitic	Rare. Usually contact lens wearers with poor hygiene, also trauma with organic material (wood, dirt, etc.)	Very severe pain	Similar to bacterial	Very difficult to diagnose, requires ophthalmologist	Will be initiated by ophthalmologist
UV	Usually related to occupation (welding) or hobbies (snow or water sports)	Severe pain within 6–12 h of exposure	• Diffuse punctate keratopathy • Corneal edema	Diagnosed clinically	Supportive. Cycloplegics, analgesics. Erythromycin ointment to prevent secondary infection
Corneal abrasion	Typically have history of known trauma (can be minor)	Pain, foreign body sensation after trauma	Corneal fluorescein uptake	Diagnosed clinically (rule out retained foreign body, open globe)	Supportive. Pain control, topical antibiotic ointment for secondary infection prevention

Subconjunctival hemorrhage	May have history of trauma or Valsalva-like increase in blood pressure (coughing, sneezing, vomiting)	Usually asymptomatic	Flat-appearing blood collection under conjunctiva, can be very large	Diagnosed clinically. May check coagulation studies in anticoagulated patients	No treatment required, typically resolves in 2 weeks
Steven-Johnson syndrome/toxic epidermal necrolysis	• Severe dermatologic condition effecting mucous membranes and skin. Typically related to drugs (antiepileptics, antibiotics)	• Rash/skin sloughing • Oral pain Nausea, vomiting	• Epidermal and mucous membrane sloughing • May seen conjunctivitis, corneal ulcers, eyelid involvement • Ocular involvement in 50–88% of cases	• Clinically diagnosed, fluorescein and slit lamp exam to evaluated ocular involvement	Admission to burn unit, emergent ophthalmology consult for ocular involvement

(continued)

TABLE 6.1 (continued)

Disease	General info	Symptoms	Physical findings	Testing indicated	Treatment
Iritis	Typical causes: • Autoimmune: Inflammatory bowel syndrome, Behcet's syndrome, etc. • Associated with an ocular infection such as keratitis • Posttraumatic • Idiopathic	• Pain, photophobia	• Consensual photophobia • Conjunctival injection with perilimbic predominance (ciliary flush) • Affected pupil may be miotic, sluggish	• Fluorescein exam Slit lamp exam – will see cell and flare	Cycloplegics, ophthalmology follow-up
Chemical burn	• Typically have known chemical exposure. Alkali typically worse than acidic exposures	Severe pain	• Blepharospasm • Conjunctival injection • May appear white in severe cases (vasospasm)	• pH testing, visual acuity – after copious irrigation	Immediate copious irrigation with isotonic solution (normal saline, lactated ringers, etc.) until pH returns to normal. Emergent ophthalmology consult

References

1. Azari AA, Barney NP. Conjunctivitis: a systematic review of diagnosis and treatment. JAMA. 2013;310(16):1721–9. https://doi.org/10.1001/jama.2013.280318.
2. Geloneck M, Binenbaum G. Conjunctivitis of the newborn. In: Lambert SR, Lyons CJ, editors. Taylor and Hoyt's pediatric ophthalmology and strabismus. 5th ed. London: Elsevier; 2017. p. 109–12.
3. Kircher J, Dixon A. Eye emergencies in infants and children. In: Tintinalli JE, Stephan Stapczynski J, John Ma O, Yealy DM, Meckler GD, Cline DM, editors. Tintinalli's emergency medicine: a comprehensive study guide. 8th ed. New York: McGraw-Hill Education; 2016. p. 770–3.
4. Rose PW, Harnden A, Brueggemann AB, et al. Chloramphenicol treatment for acute infective conjunctivitis in children in primary care: a randomised double-blind placebo-controlled trial. Lancet. 2005;366(9479):37–43. https://doi.org/10.1016/S0140-6736(05)66709-8.
5. Buznach N, Dagan R, Greenberg D. Clinical and bacterial characteristics of acute bacterial conjunctivitis in children in the antibiotic resistance era. Pediatr Infect Dis J. 2005;24(9):823–8. https://doi.org/10.1097/01.inf.0000178066.24569.98.
6. Rietveld RP, ter Riet G, Bindels PJE, Sloos JH, van Weert HCPM. Predicting bacterial cause in infectious conjunctivitis: cohort study on informativeness of combinations of signs and symptoms. BMJ. 2004;329(7459):206–10. https://doi.org/10.1136/bmj.38128.631319.AE.
7. Sheikh A, Hurwitz B. Antibiotics versus placebo for acute bacterial conjunctivitis. Cochrane Database Syst Rev. 2006;2:CD001211. https://doi.org/10.1002/14651858.CD001211.pub2.
8. Cronau H, Kankanala RR, Mauger T. Diagnosis and management of red eye in primary care. Am Fam Physician. 2010;81(2):137–45.
9. Burns JC, Glode MP. Kawasaki syndrome. Lancet. 2004;364(9433):533–44. https://doi.org/10.1016/s0140-6736(04)16814-1.
10. Ohno S, Miyajima T, Higuchi M, et al. Ocular manifestations of Kawasaki's disease (mucocutaneous lymph node syndrome). Am J Ophthalmol. 1982;93(6):713–7. http://www.ncbi.nlm.nih.gov/pubmed/7201245.

11. Carter JD, Hudson AP. Reactive arthritis: clinical aspects and medical management. Rheum Dis Clin N Am. 2009;35(1):21–44. https://doi.org/10.1016/j.rdc.2009.03.010.

12. Kvien TK, Gaston JSH, Bardin T, et al. Three month treatment of reactive arthritis with azithromycin: a EULAR double blind, placebo controlled study. Ann Rheum Dis. 2004;63(9):1113–9. https://doi.org/10.1136/ard.2003.010710.

13. Barber CE, Kim J, Inman RD, Esdaile JM, James MT. Antibiotics for treatment of reactive arthritis: a systematic review and meta-analysis. J Rheumatol. 2013;40(6):916–28. https://doi.org/10.3899/jrheum.121192.

14. Collier SA, Gronostaj MP, MacGurn AK, et al. Estimated burden of keratitis – United States, 2010. MMWR Morb Mortal Wkly Rep. 2014;63(45):1027–30.

15. Walker RA, Adhikari S. Eye emergencies. In: Tintinalli's emergency medicine: a comprehensive study guide. 8th ed. New York: McGraw-Hill Education; 2016. p. 1543–78.

16. Keenan JD, Mcleod SD. 4.12 — bacterial keratitis. 4th ed. Philadelphia: Elsevier; 2016. https://doi.org/10.1016/B978-1-4557-3984-4.00121-4.

17. Tuli SS, Kubal AA. 4.15 — herpes simplex keratitis. 4th ed. Philadelphia: Elsevier; 2016. https://doi.org/10.1016/B978-1-4557-3984-4.00124-X.

18. Wilhelmus KR. Antiviral treatment and other therapeutic interventions for herpes simplex virus epithelial keratitis. Cochrane Database Syst Rev. 2015;1(12):CD002898. https://doi.org/10.1002/14651858.CD002898.pub5.

19. Barron BA, Beck RW, Asbell PA, Cohen EJ, Dawson CR, Hyndiuk RA, Jones DB, Kaufman HE, Kurinij N, Moke PS, Doyle Stulting R, Sugar J, Wilhelmus KR. A controlled trial of oral acyclovir for the prevention of stromal keratitis or iritis in patients with herpes simplex virus epithelial keratitis. The epithelial keratitis trial. The Herpetic Eye Disease Study Group. Arch Ophthalmol (Chicago, Ill 1960). 1997;115(6):703–12. https://doi.org/10.16373/j.cnki.ahr.150049.

20. Barron BA, Gee L, Hauck WW, et al. Herpetic eye disease study. Ophthalmology. 1994;101(12):1871–82. https://doi.org/10.1016/S0161-6420(13)31155-5.

21. Vrcek I, Choudhury E, Durairaj V. Herpes zoster ophthalmicus: a review for the internist. Am J Med. 2016;130(1):21–6. https://doi.org/10.1016/j.amjmed.2016.08.039.

22. Han Y, Zhang J, Chen N, He L, Zhou M, Zhu C. Corticosteroids for preventing postherpetic neuralgia (review) summary of findings for the main comparison. 2013;3. https://doi.org/10.1002/14651858.CD005582.pub4. www.cochranelibrary.com.

23. Report MW. Adenovirus-associated epidemic keratoconjunctivitis outbreaks—four states, 2008–2010. MMWR Morb Mortal Wkly Rep. 2013;62(32):637–41.

24. Pihos AM. Epidemic keratoconjunctivitis: a review of current concepts in management. J Optom. 2013;6(2):69–74. https://doi.org/10.1016/j.optom.2012.08.003.

25. Dart JKG, Saw VPJ, Kilvington S. Acanthamoeba keratitis: diagnosis and treatment update 2009. Am J Ophthalmol. 2009;148(4):487–499.e2. https://doi.org/10.1016/j.ajo.2009.06.009.

26. Lorenzo-morales J, Khan NA, Walochnik J. An update on acanthamoeba keratitis: diagnosis, pathogenesis and treatment. Parasite. 2015;22:10. https://doi.org/10.1051/parasite/2015010.

27. Page MA, Mathers WD. Acanthamoeba keratitis: a 12-year experience covering a wide spectrum of presentations, diagnoses, and outcomes. J Ophthalmol. 2013;2013:2–7. https://doi.org/10.1155/2013/670242.

28. Jurkunas U, Behlau I, Colby K. Fungal keratitis: changing pathogens and risk factors. Cornea. 2009;28(6):638–43. https://doi.org/10.1097/ICO.0b013e318191695b.

29. Liesegang TJ, Forster RK. Spectrum of microbial keratitis in South Florida. Am J Ophthalmol. 1980;90(1):38–47. http://www.ncbi.nlm.nih.gov/pubmed/7395957.

30. Keenan JD, Mcleod SD. 4.13—fungal keratitis. 4th ed. Philadelphia: Elsevier; 2016. https://doi.org/10.1016/B978-1-4557-3984-4.00122-6.

31. Thomas PA. Fungal infections of the cornea. Eye (Lond). 2003;17(8):852–62. https://doi.org/10.1038/sj.eye.6700557.

32. Mascarenhas J, Lalitha P, Prajna NV, et al. Acanthamoeba, fungal, and bacterial keratitis: a comparison of risk factors and clinical features. Am J Ophthalmol. 2014;157(1):56–62. https://doi.org/10.1016/j.ajo.2013.08.032.

33. McIntosh SE, Guercio B, Tabin GC, Leemon D, Schimelpfenig T. Ultraviolet keratitis among mountaineers and outdoor recreationalists. Wilderness Environ Med. 2011;22(2):144–7. https://doi.org/10.1016/j.wem.2011.01.002.

34. Finn LE, Gutowski J, Alles S, et al. Photokeratitis linked to metal halide bulbs in two gymnasiums—Philadelphia, Pennsylvania, 2011 and 2013. MMWR Morb Mortal Wkly Rep. 2016;65(11):282–5. https://doi.org/10.15585/mmwr.mm6511a4.
35. Swaminathan A, Otterness K, Milne K, Rezaie S. The safety of topical anesthetics in the treatment of corneal abrasions: a review. J Emerg Med. 2015;49(5):810–5. https://doi.org/10.1016/j.jemermed.2015.06.069.
36. Calder LA, Balasubramanian S, Fergusson D. Topical nonsteroidal anti-inflammatory drugs for corneal abrasions: meta-analysis of randomized trials. Acad Emerg Med. 2005;12(5):467–73. https://doi.org/10.1197/j.aem.2004.10.026.
37. Waldman N, Densie IK, Herbison P. Topical tetracaine used for 24 hours is safe and rated highly effective by patients for the treatment of pain caused by corneal abrasions: a double-blind, randomized clinical trial. Acad Emerg Med. 2014;21(4):374–82. https://doi.org/10.1111/acem.12346.
38. Ball IM, Seabrook J, Desai N, Allen L, Anderson S. Dilute proparacaine for the management of acute corneal injuries in the emergency department. Can J Emerg Med. 2010;12(5):389–94.
39. Upadhyay MP, Karmacharya PC, Koirala S, et al. The Bhaktapur eye study: ocular trauma and antibiotic prophylaxis for the prevention of corneal ulceration in Nepal. Br J Ophthalmol. 2001;85(4):388–92. https://doi.org/10.1136/bjo.85.4.388.
40. Lim CHL, Turner A, Lim BX. Patching for corneal abrasion. Cochrane Database Syst Rev. 2016;2016(7):10–3. https://doi.org/10.1002/14651858.CD004764.pub3.
41. Wilson SA, Last A. Management of corneal abrasions. Am Fam Physician. 2004;70(1):123–30.
42. Brahma AK, Shah S, Hillier VF, et al. Topical analgesia for superficial corneal injuries. J Accid Emerg Med. 1996;13(3):186–8. https://doi.org/10.1136/emj.13.3.186.
43. Hu DN, Mou CH, Chao SC, et al. Incidence of non-traumatic subconjunctival hemorrhage in a nationwide study in Taiwan from 2000 to 2011. PLoS One. 2015;10(7):1–10. https://doi.org/10.1371/journal.pone.0132762.
44. Tarlan B, Kiratli H. Subconjunctival hemorrhage: risk factors and potential indicators. Clin Ophthalmol. 2013;7:1163–70. https://doi.org/10.2147/OPTH.S35062.
45. Sotozono C, Ueta M, Koizumi N, et al. Diagnosis and treatment of Stevens-Johnson syndrome and toxic epidermal necrolysis with ocular complications. Ophthalmology. 2009;116(4):685–90. https://doi.org/10.1016/j.ophtha.2008.12.048.

46. Kohanim S, Palioura S, Saeed HN, et al. Stevens-Johnson syndrome/toxic epidermal Necrolysis – a comprehensive review and guide to therapy. I. Systemic disease. Ocul Surf. 2016;14(1):2–19. https://doi.org/10.1016/j.jtos.2015.10.002.

47. Kohanim S, Palioura S, Saeed HN, et al. Acute and chronic ophthalmic involvement in Stevens-Johnson syndrome/toxic epidermal necrolysis – a comprehensive review and guide to therapy. II. Ophthalmic disease. Ocul Surf. 2016;14(2):168–88. https://doi.org/10.1016/j.jtos.2016.02.001.

48. Gritz DC, Wong IG. Incidence and prevalence of uveitis in northern California: the northern California epidemiology of uveitis study. Ophthalmology. 2004;111(3):491–500. https://doi.org/10.1016/j.ophtha.2003.06.014.

49. Suhler EB, Lloyd MJ, Choi D, Rosenbaum JT, Austin DF. Incidence and prevalence of uveitis in veterans affairs medical centers of the Pacific northwest. Am J Ophthalmol. 2008;146(6):890–6. https://doi.org/10.1016/j.ajo.2008.09.014.

50. Acharya NR, Tham VM, Esterberg E, et al. Incidence and prevalence of uveitis. JAMA Ophthalmol. 2013;131(11):1405. https://doi.org/10.1001/jamaophthalmol.2013.4237.

51. Read R. General approach to the uveitis patient and treatment strategies. In: Yanoff M, editor. Ophthalmology. 4th ed. Philadelphia: Elsevier; 2014. p. 694–9.

52. Suttorp-Schulten MS, Rothova A. The possible impact of uveitis in blindness: a literature survey. Br J Ophthalmol. 1996;80(9):844–8. https://doi.org/10.1136/bjo.80.9.844.

53. McCannel CA, Holland GN, Helm CJ, et al. Causes of uveitis in the general practice of ophthalmology. Am J Ophthalmol. 1996;121(1):35–46. https://doi.org/10.1016/S0002-9394(14)70532-X.

54. Herr RD, White GL, Bernhisel K, Mamalis N, Swanson E. Clinical comparison of ocular irrigation fluids following chemical injury. Am J Emerg Med. 1991;9(3):228–31. http://www.ncbi.nlm.nih.gov/pubmed/1850282

55. Fish R, Davidson RS. Management of ocular thermal and chemical injuries, including amniotic membrane therapy. Curr Opin Ophthalmol. 2010;21(4):317–21. https://doi.org/10.1097/ICU.0b013e32833a8da2.

56. Spector J, Fernandez WG. Chemical, thermal, and biological ocular exposures. Emerg Med Clin North Am. 2008;26(1):125–36. https://doi.org/10.1016/j.emc.2007.11.002.

Chapter 7
Painful Eye

Natalie Sciano

Brief Introduction

The painful eye carries a wide differential from self-limiting etiologies to those that are vision threatening. A painful eye can be very distressing to a patient, not only due to pain but from the fear of vision loss. Common themes throughout the treatment of a painful eye include controlling pain, decreasing inflammation, and preventing subsequent complication such as infection and scarring which can lead to lasting visual impairments. Additionally, some patients may require a multidisciplinary approach necessitating multiple specialty referrals depending on history and examination findings. Therefore, when confronted with the painful eye, the emergency physician must consider the etiologies discussed below, attempt to alleviate the patient's pain and fears, and recognize those needing further workup to improve patient outcomes.

N. Sciano, MD
Emergency Department, University of Texas Southwestern Medical Center, Dallas, TX, USA

© Springer International Publishing AG, part of Springer Nature 2018
B. Long, A. Koyfman (eds.), *Handbook of Emergency Ophthalmology*, https://doi.org/10.1007/978-3-319-78945-3_7

Clinical Presentation

Patients presenting with a painful eye may simply report pain to the eye, which is more often unilateral. It could be acute in onset or even indolent. Additional complaints that often accompany pain include photophobia, tearing, itching, and foreign body sensation. Keep in mind that eye pain may not simply be an ocular cause. It can be referred pain from the sinuses or even a neurological condition.

Differential Diagnosis

The differential diagnosis for painful eye is quite broad. It includes keratitis, corneal abrasion, corneal ulcer, uveitis, episcleritis, scleritis, acute angle closure glaucoma (AACG), conjunctivitis, temporal arteritis or giant cell arteritis, optic neuritis, ocular migraine, cavernous sinus thrombosis, trigeminal neuralgia, orbital cellulitis, sinusitis, and others. Differentiating etiologies involves determining if the eye pain is solely ocular in origin, is this referred pain, or is there a larger systemic process involved.

Clinical Evaluation

The history can be extremely helpful in determining the etiology of a painful eye. Helpful discussion topics with the patient include acuity in onset, trauma history, prior episodes, immune status such as HIV or steroid use, work environment, eye history including prior surgeries or contact use, and medication history. Some examples of helpful questions with differentials are listed in Table 7.1.

After the history, a physical examination provides further essential information to the emergency physician for assistance with diagnosis and treatment. In addition, to a complete ocular examination, special attention should be taken on the neurological, musculoskeletal, and dermatological examina-

TABLE 7.1 Clinical evaluation

Example of questions to ask	Differential diagnosis examples
History of the present illness	
Was the pain acute in onset or progressive?	AACG, traumatic, infection
Was there trauma involved? If so, was it blunt or penetrating?	Globe injury, traumatic iritis
Chemical exposure?	Corneal abrasion, burns
Is it bilateral?	Keratitis, conjunctivitis
Is there vision loss or vision impairment?	AACG, optic neuritis, uveitis, temporal arteritis
Is there fever associated with other symptoms?	Systemic infection, orbital cellulitis
Is the pain worse with eye movement?	Optic neuritis, orbital cellulitis
Is there a history of neurological symptoms?	Optic neuritis, rheumatologic
Is there a rash?	Infections, rheumatologic
Recent travel history including travel to endemic areas	Infections, keratitis
(Lyme, histoplasmosis, etc.), sun exposure, etc.? [1]	
Work exposure?	Chemical burns, UV keratitis
Past medical history	
Do you wear contacts? If so, how often do you exchange them?	Ulcers, abrasions, uveitis, keratitis
History of cold sores/HSV, chicken pox, HIV	Ulcers, zoster ophthalmicus
Syphilis, tuberculosis?	

(continued)

TABLE 7.1 (continued)

Example of questions to ask	Differential diagnosis examples
Medication history	
Do you use eye drops, specifically topical steroid gtts?	Infection
Are you on immunosuppressants?	Infection, rheumatologic
Is the patient taking anticholinergic, sympathomimetic, or sulfa drugs? [2]	AACG
Family history	
Other family members with similar conditions?	AACG

tions when pertinent. Tetanus should always be updated when necessary. Except for chemical burns, which require immediate irrigation prior to examination, the following examination steps can be taken in a patient presenting with a painful eye [3]:

1. Visual acuity: This could be seen as the vital sign of the eye, when a patient presents with any ocular complaint. This ideally can be taken before a patient is seen by a provider. Each eye is assessed separately and together. The line at which the patient can read half of the letters correctly is the visual acuity.
2. Extraocular movements: Assess the cranial nerves' function. If there is pain with movements, one may be concerned for optic neuritis or orbital cellulitis.
3. External examination: This includes assessment of eyelids, eyelashes, conjunctiva, and sclera.
4. Pupils: Determine the pupils' shape, equality to each other, reaction to light, presence of pain with light, and presence of an afferent pupillary defect.
5. Pressure: Measure intraocular pressure of each eye after applying topical anesthetic (tetracaine). Normal intraocular pressure is <20 mmHg. Make sure not to put pressure

accidently on the globe while opening the eye, which can cause errors in measurements.

6. Slit-lamp examination: This can be used to assess the anterior chamber of an eye for cell flare which can be seen in various etiologies as discussed later. Hypopyon and hyphema will also be better visualized if small. Additionally, closer inspection of conjunctiva and sclera with the slit lamp is possible.

7. Wood's lamp examination or cobalt blue filter: Instill the eye with fluorescein to assess for corneal defects such as abrasions and ulcers. To introduce fluorescein into the eye, first apply eye solution to the fluorescein strip. Then apply fluorescein into the eye at the inferior conjunctival fornix. This will hopefully prevent a linear striping of the fluorescein, which can be confused with an abrasion.

Clinical Conditions and Management

Keratitis

Keratitis is inflammation of the cornea. The cornea is an avascular structure and has five anatomical layers from anterior to posterior: epithelium, Bowman's layer, corneal stroma, Descemet's membrane, and the endothelium. Keratitis can have an infectious or noninfectious etiology which includes exposure, dry eyes, and drug induced. It is most often bilateral with common complaints including pain, foreign body sensation, photophobia, and tearing. The cornea contains many sensory nerves so pain can be quite intense. Complications of keratitis include ulceration, perforation, scarring leading to vision loss, glaucoma, or uveitis [4, 5].

If only the epithelial layer is involved, it is termed superficial punctate keratitis (SPK). This process will demonstrate scattered pinpoint uptake of fluorescence on Wood's lamp or slit-lamp examination. Depending on the etiology, these foci of uptake may be scattered or located centrally, superiorly, or inferiorly on the cornea. A classic example is UV keratitis caused by prolonged UV ray exposure such as welding professionals or prolonged sun exposure from skiing without eye protection. The pain typically occurs 6–12 h after exposure, so a patient may wake up the next day with symptoms [4, 6]. Treatment involves topical lubricants such as erythromycin and artificial tears. Adding cycloplegics will help decrease ciliary spasm [6, 7]. These lesions usually heal within 48–72 h without sequelae.

Infectious keratitis can occur from bacteria, viruses, fungi, or amoebae. The incidence of bacterial keratitis has increased with the use of contacts [4]. Additionally, the culprit organism has evolved from *Streptococcus pneumoniae* to *Pseudomonas*, *Staphylococcus*, and *Serratia* as contact lens wearing increases. Physical examination will reveal a corneal infiltrate with fluorescein uptake and sometimes a hypopyon and cell and flare on anterior chamber examination, which are more common in pseudomonal infections [4, 6]. These findings are especially worrisome due *Pseudomonas'* rapid corneal destruction which can lead to entire corneal involvement, ulceration, and possible perforation [4, 5]. Topical antibiotics are the treatment of choice with tailoring based on most likely organism. Same-day ophthalmology referral or admission may be required based on the patient's ability to comply, social circumstances, or follow-up ability [4, 6].

Chlamydial keratitis can occur with any of the chlamydial infections including trachoma, lymphogranuloma venereum, and psittacosis. The incubation period ranges from 5 to 14 days. Keratitis with superficial punctate lesions usually involves the upper third of the cornea [5]. Keratitis findings can be associated with conjunctivitis. These patients will have minimal itching and exudates, usually without fever or sore throat [8]. Exudates may cause eyelids to be stuck together upon awaking. Trachoma can cause chronic follicular conjunctivitis that leads to conjunctival scarring, inturned lashes (trichiasis), and defective tearing leading to corneal scarring, ulceration, and vision loss. Treatment involves oral or topical agents such as erythromycin, sulfonamide, or tetracycline ointments that are used QID for 6 weeks. Systemic therapy involves doxycycline (100 mg BID for 3 weeks), erythromycin (1 g/day QID for 3–4 weeks), or tetracycline (1 g per day QID for 3–4 weeks). Do not use tetracycline in children under 7 years old [5].

Viral keratitis etiologies include HSV, VZV, EBV, and adenovirus. HSV, the most common form, and VZV will be discussed in the section on corneal ulcers [6]. Adenovirus will cause preauricular lymphadenopathy, bilateral conjunctivitis, and painful red eye. Pharyngitis or gastrointestinal complaints may also be present. It usually reaches its peak at 5–7 days [5]. The epidemic form, lay term pink eye, is caused by adenovirus types 8 and 19. Topical steroids can make the patient more comfortable but may prolong the disease. Consultation with an ophthalmologist prior to starting steroids is recommended. Fluorescein examination may show fine or small scattered erosions.

Drug-induced epithelial keratitis is also possible. Toxic substances include the aminoglycosides and topical antiviral agents [5]. Neurotrophic keratitis is caused by recurrent corneal injury due to decreased sensation of the cornea [4, 5]. Without the ability to sense pain, these patients must be vigilant to redness, discharge, and vision changes, signs of inflammatory and infectious processes. The goal is eye lubrication and treatment of the underlying condition. Exposure keratitis is related to incomplete closure of the eyelid such as in Bell's palsy, ectropion, and exophthalmos. The treatment is lubrication with possible nightly eye protection such as swim goggles [5, 6].

Another entity that may be encountered is keratoconjunctivitis sicca. These lesions will be filamentous and usually in the lower half of the cornea [5]. The lesions are due to dry eyes from decreased lubricant production from the lacrimal and accessory glands. This may be due to Sjogren's syndrome, which is an inflammatory condition resulting in infiltration of exocrine organs. Patients may present with xerophthalmia (dry eyes), xerostomia (dry mouth), and parotid gland enlargement [9]. The treatment aims at replacing the lost lubrication with use of tear substitutes and lubricating ointments. Swim goggles may be used at night to entrap the moisture [5].

Corneal Ulcer

Ulcerative keratitis involves inflammation of the epithelial layer producing significant erosion with ultimate formation of an epithelial defect or ulcer. Ulcers can be infectious but can be seen in many rheumatological condition such as rheumatoid arthritis, sarcoid, and other vasculitides. A major complication of corneal ulceration involves the process of cicatrization which is the production of a corneal scar leading to visual defects [4, 5]. Patients need ophthalmology consultation and follow-up within 24 h [6].

An infectious ulcer is usually within the central cornea and can be accompanied by hypopyon and anterior uveitis if severe. Prior to the surge in contact lens use, *Streptococcus pneumoniae* was the usual culprit. These ulcers were usually due to a complication of trauma to the cornea. Patients infected with *S. pneumoniae* may also present with concomitant dacryocystitis and nasolacrimal duct obstruction. Now *Pseudomonas* and even the protozoa, *Acanthamoeba*, are becoming more prevalent due to contact lens wearers [5, 6].

Pseudomonas, a gram-negative rod, produces ulcers that begin as a gray or yellow corneal infiltrate which quickly progress. The eye may even have a bluish-green exudate due to the pigment produced by these organisms. A hypopyon can be present. As discussed previously, these infectious are most often due to extended contact lens use. Severe consequences including corneal perforation with seeding of the anterior chamber causing an intraocular infection are possible. Treatment involves the use of antipseudomonal agents including moxifloxacin, tobramycin, ciprofloxacin, and gentamicin [5].

Moraxella liquefaciens is becoming recognized as a common cause of corneal ulcers in alcoholics due to the pyridoxine deficiency. This is also a causative organism in diabetics and other immunosuppressed states. Treatment of the gram-negative rod involves fluoroquinolone ophthalmologic drops [5].

If practicing within an agricultural setting, be aware of fungal keratitis. Fungal keratitis can be due to *Fusarium* and *Aspergillus* from vegetable matter. *Candida* may be the underlying organism in patients with a past medical history of ocular disease. The distinction is often made after results from a corneal epithelium scraping by the ophthalmologist, so these are usually treated at first presentation as bacterial keratitis. These ulcers are often irregular, caused significant ocular inflammation, and produce satellite lesions. Treatment options include amphotericin B, voriconazole, or posaconazole, but again this entity is usual diagnosed in cultures [4, 5].

Acanthamoeba is a protozoan that can cause infection in contact lens wearers or those exposed to contaminated water. Typically there is pain out of proportion to examination findings with accompanied redness and photophobia [5]. Dendritic-like lesions may be seen on slit-lamp examination, so this diagnosis can be confused with HSV keratitis. If suspected due to history and physical examination, prompt referral should be initiated, as biopsy and culture are required for diagnosis. These patients may be started on topical propamidine isethionate (1% solution) and fortified neomycin drops [4, 5].

As discussed previously, HSV keratitis involves the replication of the herpes simplex virus within the corneal epithelium. HSV is the most common cause of corneal ulcers in the United States [10]. Infections are most commonly due to HSV type 1 [4, 5, 10]. After a primary dermatological infection with HSV, the virus will lay dormant within the trigeminal ganglion. Keratitis may then develop 1–2 weeks after the appearance of the primary skin infection. The classic lesion is a unilateral, dendritic-appearing corneal defect. It can progress and enlarge to form a geographic ulcer [10]. The classic dendritic lesion of linear branching and terminal bulbs coalesce to form a larger geographic ulcer. It recurs in 25–30% of patients within 2 years with triggers being surgery, trauma, menstrual cycle, or stress [4, 5, 10].

Most herpetic lesions will resolve in a couple weeks with or without therapy. However, therapy is indicated to help reduce the risk of corneal scarring. Topical antiviral therapy includes trifluridine 1% drops (q3–4 h/8× per day) or vidarabine 3% ointment (5× per day). If a geographic ulcer is present, trifluridine is more effective [10]. Topical antiviral ocular toxicity can occur, so prompt ophthalmologic follow-up is indicated to taper or discontinue these medications depending on ulcer healing [5, 10]. Adjuncts include oral acyclovir (400 mg five times per day, 2 g/day) [10]. Topical steroids should be avoided. Ophthalmologists may also decide to debride the lesions to decrease the corneal viral load [5] (Table 7.2).

Varicella zoster virus (VZV) can be a primary or recurrent infection. The primary infection is due to varicella skin infection, also known as chicken pox. The recurrent infection is confusingly termed herpes zoster or shingles. Specifically, herpes zoster can have ocular manifestation termed ophthalmic zoster or herpes zoster ophthalmicus. Though chicken pox can be present on the eyelid or lid margins, it rarely

TABLE 7.2 Viral ulcer treatment

Treatment options for herpes simplex keratitis/ulcers	
Antiviral	Dosing
Topical trifluridine 1% solution	Every 3–4 h or 8× per day
Topical vidarabine 3% ointment	5× per day
Adjunct oral acyclovir	2 g per day
Treatment options for zoster ophthalmicus	
Oral acyclovir	800 mg 5× per day 10–14 days
Oral famciclovir	500 mg TID 7–10 days
Oral valacyclovir	1 g TID 7–10 days
Analgesia	NSAIDs
Prophylactic antibiotics	Erythromycin ointment
Decreased eyelid function	Artificial tears

involves the globe itself [5]. If the nasociliary branch of the trigeminal nerve is involved, ocular manifestations are more likely. With involvement of the nasociliary branch, the classic finding is skin vesicles at the tip of the nose termed Hutchinson's sign [5]. VZV can cause decreased corneal sensation leading to less pain than anticipated. Additionally, this virus more commonly infects the stromal layer and anterior uveal structures, compared to HSV [4, 5, 10]. The classic pattern is pseudodendritic, which can be confused with HSV keratitis [10]. Treatment is similar to HSV and involves oral acyclovir (800 mg 5×/day for 7–10 days) or valacyclovir (1 g TID for 7–10 days). This should be ideally started within 3 days of skin lesions [4, 5, 10]. Wound care and antibiotic prophylaxis for secondary bacterial infection are commonly prescribed. If blinking is impaired, eye lubricant should be provided to prevent desiccation [10]. Treatment does not prevent the development of postherpetic neuralgia, unfortunately [5].

Corneal Abrasion

Corneal abrasions are one of the most common eye-related complaints presenting to the emergency department [11, 12]. An abrasion is a defect within the corneal epithelium usually resulting from trauma, foreign bodies, contact lenses, and flash burns [4, 12]. The corneal epithelium is the first layer of the cornea, which can regenerate quickly and is not involved in the corneal dehydration process, so damage is only transient. The cornea is made up of many pain-sensing fibers causing the patient significant pain, photophobia, and tearing [5]. Treatment involves decreasing pain, preventing infection, and allowing healing of the defect. However, the treatment regimen is often subjective and based on physician preference, typically including oral analgesics, topical analgesics, cycloplegics, or a combination.

Utilize a short-acting topical anesthetic, such as tetracaine or proparacaine, to decrease pain in order to further analyze the eye. On physical examination, if there is significant edema, visual acuity may be impaired. The pupil may be miotic due to ciliary spasm, and the patient's eyelid may have blepharospasm due to severe photophobia [4]. The defect is visualized using fluorescein and a Wood's lamp or cobalt filter light. Keep in mind that if the defects are linear and vertically oriented, there may be a foreign body within the eyelid. Eversion of eyelids should be done when this is suspected. More severe pathology such as intraocular injury should always be on the differential especially if projectiles or metal work is involved. After fluorescein is applied, Seidel sign may be present. Seidel is the presence of flowing fluorescent aqueous humor from an intraocular globe injury and is an ophthalmologic emergency [6]. This is in stark contrast to the simple uptake from an abrasion.

To decrease pain, cycloplegics are utilized to decrease ciliary spasm. There is no need to patch the eye. Contacts should not be worn until healing has completed and symptoms resolved. Oral analgesics can be used for pain control [4]. Though expensive, topical NSAIDS may be an option in the right patient. These have been shown to decrease pain without the risk of infection, and patients may return to work earlier [4]. Healing occurs within a couple days. Refer to an ophthalmologist for large abrasions, contact wearers, those who develop ulcers, and those with continued pain after several days.

Corneal abrasions, unless complicated, heal within 72 h, so long-term topical anesthetic use is unnecessary. The fear of outpatient topical anesthetics has stemmed from the idea of delayed healing leading to corneal ulceration and direct corneal toxicity with prolonged use. These theories are based on case reports, case series, and animal studies. Due to this fear, however, there continues to be a lack of large studies [12]. A recent review analyzed the literature available, and it appears dilute topical anesthetics (e.g., 0.05% proparacaine) may be used safely for up to a week for corneal abrasions with close ophthalmologic follow-up [11, 13] (Table 7.3).

TABLE 7.3 Medications for corneal abrasions

Cycloplegics	Reduce pain, photophobia by decreasing ciliary spasm	Cyclopentolate ophthalmic (1%) 1 gtt every 6–8 h Homatropine ophthalmic (5%) 1–2 gtts BID
Antibiotics – Ointments – Drops (gtts)	Contact lens wearers need pseudomonal coverage	Ciprofloxacin ophthalmic (0.3%) 1–2 gtts every 2–4 h Others: tobramycin, gentamicin, ofloxacin
	Noncontact lens wearers	Erythromycin ointment apply 1 cm QID
Topical NSAIDs	Decrease pain, expensive	Topical diclofenac, ketorolac

Acute Angle Closure Glaucoma

Acute angle closure glaucoma (AACG) is an acute increase in intraocular pressure due to blockage of aqueous circulation or pupillary blockage preventing flow leading to vascular and nerve compromise [14]. This is a vision-threatening disorder. It is an anatomical dysfunction, and there is often a hereditary predisposition putting first-degree relatives of those with AACG at increased risk [4, 14]. Acute angle closure glaucoma more commonly involves individuals with hyperopia (farsightedness), women (2:1 to 4:1), and Eskimo and Asian ethnicities [4, 14]. African Americans with acute angle closure glaucoma are rare; however, African Americans often report fewer symptoms and less pain so the incidence may actually be underreported. The incidence increases with age, with the peak incidence during ages 60–70 years [15].

Any mechanism causing dilation of the pupil could potentially cause acute angle closure glaucoma including dimly lit rooms (classically movie theaters), topical mydriatics,

TABLE 7.4 Causes of acute angle closure glaucoma

Dimly lit room, e.g., movie theaters	Anticholinergics
Topical mydriatics	Tricyclic antidepressants
Selective serotonin reuptake inhibitors	Adrenergic agonists

anticholinergics, tricyclic antidepressants, selective serotonin reuptake inhibitors, or adrenergic agonists (see Table 7.4). Acute angle closure glaucoma is most commonly unilateral, but if medications are the culprit, bilateral symptoms may occur [4].

Symptoms include an acutely painful eye that is red with associated blurry vision and halos around lights [14]. Headache, nausea, and vomiting can also be present. In any patient with headache, acute angle closure glaucoma should be on the differential with adequate pupillary assessment on physical examination. The patient may describe frequent nighttime headaches due to the pupillary dilation mechanisms until finally an acute angle closure glaucoma develops.

On physical examination, the conjunctiva will be injected with mid-dilated and fixed pupil. The cornea may exhibit clouding, leading to the patient's complaints of impaired or blurry vision [4, 14, 15]. Intraocular pressure will be elevated above 20 mmHg, often between 40 and 90 mmHg [15]. One may perform the oblique flashlight test, which involves shining a light parallel, from lateral to medial, at the iris in order to evaluate the anterior chamber. A narrow anterior chamber predisposes to acute angle glaucoma. A positive test will reveal shadowing of the medial iris or nasal iris.

Once recognized, reduction of the intraocular pressure must commence to preserve the patient's vision. Prolonged intraocular pressures can lead to optic nerve atrophy and permanent vision loss. Agents used to lower intraocular pressure include topical alpha-two agonists, topical beta-blockers, and carbonic anhydrase inhibitors (see Table 7.5). If no contraindications exist, the initial regimen recommended by the AOA (American Optometric Association) to control an acute angle closure glaucoma attack includes [15]:

TABLE 7.5 Medications for acute angle glaucoma

Type	Dosing	Considerations
Topical alpha-two agonists	Apraclonidine 1% 1–2 gtt initially, repeated at 1 h if necessary	
Topical beta-blockers	Timolol 0.5% 1 gtt initially, repeated at 1 h if necessary	Caution in asthmatic, cardiac history
Carbonic anhydrase inhibitors	Acetazolamide 500 mg PO or IV	Contraindicated in patients with sulfa allergy
Topical miotic	Pilocarpine 2% 1 gtt q15–60 min to a total of four doses	Helpful once IOP <50 mmHg; caution in elderly for cholinergic crisis
Hyperosmotic	Mannitol 20% solution of 2.5–10 mL/kg IV	Caution in elderly and those that are dehydrated; risk of pulmonary edema
Topical steroids	Prednisolone 1% QID	

1. Apraclonidine 1% 1 gtt
2. Timolol 0.5% 1 gtt
3. Pilocarpine 2% 1 gtt
4. Acetazolamide 500 mg PO

Intraocular pressure should be checked every 15–30 min. If no relief of elevated pressures at 1 h, a hyperosmotic agent should be provided. Once an attack is resolved, which is defined by normal intraocular pressure, miotic pupil, and an open angle, the patient should be maintained on pilocarpine 2% QID bilaterally until follow-up. Bilateral treatment is initiated due to AACG's anatomical risk factors [15]. If untreated, the other eye possesses a 40–80% of developing AACG within 5–10 years [14]. Topical steroids such as prednisolone can be initiated after acute angle glaucoma has been treated to inhibit the inflammation, but only after the acute incident.

Iritis/Uveitis

The uveal tract consists of the three parts: the choroid, ciliary body, and the iris. Inflammation of any of these structures is termed uveitis. Uveitis can be broken down into spatial classification including anterior, intermediate, posterior, and diffuse or panuveitis. The term anterior uveitis involves the anterior structures: ciliary body and iris. Terminology for specific areas of anterior inflammation includes cyclitis (ciliary body), iritis (iris), or iridocyclitis (iritis and ciliary body). Anterior uveitis, iritis, and iridocyclitis are often used interchangeably [1].

Anterior uveitis occurs in people ages 20–50 years old, peaking in the third decade [1, 4, 16]. Disease less than 6 weeks is acute, while that greater than 6 weeks is chronic [1]. Anterior uveitis can be idiopathic, traumatic, infectious, or associated with systemic disorders. Anterior uveitis is idiopathic in 60% of cases [4]. Traumatic anterior uveitis is usually due to blunt trauma. It is more common in developing countries due to infectious causes such as tuberculosis and toxoplasmosis [16]. Overall, many infectious etiologies are possible including but not limited to syphilis, Lyme, HSV, VZV, and CMV, as well as malignancy including leukemia, lymphoma, retinoblastoma, and melanoma [4, 16]. If syphilis is the culprit, it should be treated at neurosyphilis [4]. In HIV patients, the antibiotics rifabutin and the antiviral cidofovir are also culprits [17]. The HLA-B27 phenotype predominates in North America and Europe [4]. Patients with systemic conditions including juvenile rheumatoid arthritis, sarcoidosis, and the seronegative arthropathies—psoriatic arthritis, ankylosing spondylitis (AS), reactive arthritis (formerly Reiter's), and inflammatory bowel disease conditions—can also develop anterior uveitis. Fifty percent of those with AS will develop anterior uveitis [16]. Though rare, Behcet's disease is seen in adult males of Mediterranean and Japanese descent with the classic triad of mouth ulcers, genital ulcers, and anterior uveitis [1].

Anterior uveitis is the most common form of uveal tract inflammation. Pain, photophobia, and blurred vision are common [4, 16]. It is most often unilateral [6, 16]. Physical examination may reveal circumcorneal or limbic redness (AKA ciliary flush) with scant conjunctival injection. The pupil may be poorly reactive and constricted [6]. On slit-lamp examination, "cell and flare" representing inflammatory debris can be seen. Severe anterior uveitis may even reveal a hypopyon [4, 16]. Consensual photophobia or pain in the affected eye with light being shone in the unaffected eye is common [4]. IOP is relatively unchanged but if elevated may represent evidence of corneal edema [1]. Uveitis may be confused with conjunctivitis, keratitis, or acute angle closure glaucoma [16] (see Table 7.6).

Most cases resolve within 6 weeks. Complications of uveitis include cataracts, glaucoma, band keratopathy, and macular edema [1]. Band keratopathy is calcium deposition within the anterior cornea. Treatment involves decreasing inflammation with use of steroids and cycloplegics or mydriatics and oral anti-inflammatories. Prednisolone acetate 1% one to two drops every 1–2 h is usually recommended in conjunction with close ophthalmology or optometry follow-up [1, 4, 16]. Cycloplegics are anticholinergic agents which

Table 7.6 Uveitis differential mimics

	Findings
Uveitis	Cell flare, circumcorneal redness with minimal conjunctival and palpebral injection
Conjunctivitis	Discharge, injection of palpebral and bulbar conjunctiva
Keratitis	Stain uptake, stromal thickening, relief with topical analgesic
Acute angle closure glaucoma	Elevated IOP, corneal haze, narrow anterior chamber

inhibit the iris sphincter and ciliary muscle. Commonly used topical cycloplegics are cyclopentolate, atropine, homatropine, and scopolamine. If IOP is elevated, consider a topical beta-blocker such as timolol. A multidisciplinary approach with an additional referral to rheumatology, internist, gastroenterologist, and/or dermatologist may be warranted if a systemic disease is suspected [1, 16].

Intermediate and posterior uveitis are difficult for the emergency physician to diagnose given the nonspecific symptoms of floaters and blurry vision and, additionally, pain and redness being uncommon presentations [4, 16]. Patients with these nonspecific symptoms without acute emergent pathology should have ophthalmologic or optometric follow-up for further testing. However, caution is warranted in patients with HIV, AIDS-defining clinical conditions, and those on chemotherapy or immunosuppressants. Posterior uveitis involves the retina and choroid and can also be termed retinitis or chorioretinitis. These patients are at risk for toxoplasmosis, histoplasmosis, CMV, tuberculosis, and other infections. Cytomegalovirus (CMV) retinitis is a harbinger for severe immunosuppression with CD4 counts less than 100 cells/μL with eye complaints [17, 18]. Patient will have progressive vision loss and experience floaters and flashes. The retina may show white infiltrates and hemorrhages, which are classically described as a pizza pie [17]. Retinal detachment is a complication. Treatment involves admission for intravenous ganciclovir [18].

Optic Neuritis

Optic neuritis is the inflammation and demyelination of the optic nerve [4, 19]. It is most classically associated with multiple sclerosis but can be involved in many other disease processes including sarcoidosis, systemic lupus erythematosus, lymphoma, leukemia, and syphilis. It more commonly affects women with the median age being 30 years old [4]. The incidence is about 6.4 per 100,000, and the disease is more common in the northern latitudes [19]. The risk of developing multiple sclerosis after an episode of optic neuritis ranges from 20 to 40% [4, 6].

Patients will describe unilateral eye pain and vision loss or decreased vision with classically a change in color perception. Symptoms manifest over hours to days. The eye pain is worse with movement and is associated with an afferent pupillary defect [4, 19]. Papilledema may or may not be present [4]. Optic neuritis is a clinical diagnosis, but magnetic resonance imaging of the orbits will show enhancement at the optic nerve. These patients must be admitted to the hospital for intravenous methylprednisolone. Intravenous steroids return a patient's vision to normal more rapidly than oral steroid therapy [4, 19]. Consultation with ophthalmology and neurology is warranted.

Chemical and Thermal Burns

Chemical and thermal burns are ophthalmologic emergencies. These injuries are often workplace or household related. Alkali injuries are more common than acid injuries [3]. Alkali exposures are more severe due to a liquefactive necrosis cascade of protein denaturing and saponification of ocular tissue. Common examples of alkali are ammonia and lye. Acidic injuries are less common and cause coagulation necrosis, creating a coagulum that acts as a barrier to further damage [3, 7]. The damage incurred by alkali exposures is directly proportional to the surface area exposed and time elapsed. The most severe injuries are due to ammonia and lye, which are common household products [3, 7]. Ammonia causes injury within 1 min, and lye causes deep injury within 3–5 min. Sulfuric acid is the most common acidic injury but does not usually produce significant injury. Hydrofluoric acid (HF) is an exception to the rule for acidic burns. HF, found in rust remover, leather tanner, and high-octane gasoline, acts more like an alkali substance causing liquefactive necrosis [7].

Time is eye, and the mainstay of treatment in chemical injuries is irrigation. Even before presenting to the emergency department, irrigation should commence using tap water or any nontoxic solution available. An ocular examination should not be performed until irrigation has completed. Prepare the eye with a topical anesthetic prior to irrigation. Start with 1–2 L per eye of continuous irrigation with normal saline or an isotonic solution. Morgan lenses should be utilized when available. Assess the pH of each eye at 30 min intervals with litmus paper. Once the pH has been restored to normal, irrigation may be paused. Assess the pH one more time 30 minutes after discontinuing the irrigation. If the eyes continue to demonstrate normal pH, no further irrigation is necessary [20]. A complete ocular examination including intraocular pressure, fluorescein, anterior chamber assessment, and visual acuity should take place.

Complications of chemical injuries include corneal scarring, perforation, and vision loss. Various post-irrigation treatment modalities exist depending on the extent of injury. They could include but not limited to topical antibiotics, cycloplegics, steroids, lubricants, and acetazolamide [21]. This post-irrigation treatment should always be in conjunction with an assessment by an ophthalmologist [7, 21].

Ocular injuries also include thermal burns from fires, explosions, flash burns, or heated objects such as curling irons. Due to the corneal reflex, it is more common to see swelling, blistering, and charring of the skin rather than an ocular injury [7]. However, if present, treatment is the same as for chemical injuries. Irrigation and removal of the hot debris from the eye should be performed as quickly as possible. Additionally, these will need topical antibiotic ointment (erythromycin 0.5%) for infectious prevention as well as lubrication [7, 21]. Cycloplegics (cyclopentolate 0.5%) can also be given. Complications include ectropion, corneal desiccation, and ulceration [21].

If cyanoacrylate (i.e., super glue, crazy glue) exposure occurs, the application of a copious amount of erythromycin ointment on the lids and onto the eye is recommended. This will help loosen the glue for easier removal. Cyanoacrylate may result in irritation, causing local dermatitis or corneal abrasions [5, 7].

Episcleritis and Scleritis

The sclera is a collagenous structure extending from the cornea to the optic foramen posteriorly. The vascular connective tissue layer overlying the sclera is termed the episclera. The scleral rigidity helps provide protection and allows for a constant intraocular pressure with eye movement. Additionally, the opacity decreases internal scatter in order for the retina to obtain an adequate image. Scleritis is inflammation of the sclera and, though uncommon, should be recognized by emergency physicians due to the risk of vision loss and potential underlying systemic disease.

Scleritis has an average age of onset of 48 years old and is more common in females [4, 16]. Scleritis is more commonly from contributing immunological factors such as rheumatologic diseases. Episcleritis is usually not immunologically based. Rheumatoid arthritis is the most common culprit [4]. It is an insidious pain that grows to become intensely painful. It can have referred periocular bone pain, as well as jaw and facial pain due to cranial nerve five involvement. It can be so severe that it awakes patients from sleep [4, 16].

Anterior scleritis involves the visible portion of sclera. It can be diffuse, nodular (i.e., focal), and necrotizing. Diffuse is the most common [6]. The sclera can appear diffusely violaceous or bluish due to the edema and engorgement of the vasculature with thinning of the sclera. This is in contrast to episcleritis, which involves the superficial vessels and will not thin the sclera. Complications of anterior scleritis include thinning of the sclera, loss of opacity of the sclera, increased IOP, and even vision loss if the cornea becomes involved. Treatment involves NSAIDS such as indomethacin or ibuprofen. Urgent referral to an ophthalmologist is indicated due to the potential complications, and the patient may require topical or oral steroids [6, 16]. Postsurgical patients may even develop an aggressive form of anterior scleritis termed surgically induced necrotizing scleritis (SINS), which is an ophthalmologic emergency.

Posterior scleritis is difficult to diagnose, as this portion of the sclera is not visible. Due to this fact, it is often not diagnosed early and treated late with vision loss as a complication. It may be painful or painless. The patient could complain of vision changes due to inflammatory involvement of the nearby extraocular muscles that can cause blurry vision and diplopia. Interestingly, ultrasound can play a role in diagnosis. On ultrasound, the posterior aspects of the eye will show scleral thickening and even a fluid collection due to edema [16].

Episcleritis is the inflammation of the vascular connective tissue layer overlying the sclera, i.e., episclera. It is usually more common in women and occurs during the third and fourth decade of life. It is often acute in onset pain with the eye becoming red. It can be diffuse or nodular. Episcleritis can be diffuse or only involve a focal area of inflammation termed nodular episcleritis. Though uncomfortable for the patient, episcleritis is a benign condition compared to scleritis, lasts 1–2 weeks, and is usually unilateral [6, 16]. Recurrence is common. It is more often idiopathic but can be associated with systemic disorders like collagen-vascular diseases. Treatment can include artificial tears and topical steroids for severe cases. Discuss with an ophthalmologist before starting topical steroids.

Disposition

Emergency medicine physicians play a crucial role in the assessment and management of patients presenting with a painful red eye. Immediate treatment is required for chemical and thermal injuries even prior to examination. Emergent referral to an ophthalmologist is required for chemical and thermal burns, optic neuritis, herpes zoster ophthalmicus, corneal ulcers, and acute angle closure glaucoma. Urgent referral or evaluation within 24–48 h is needed for keratitis, corneal abrasions, uveitis, scleritis, and episcleritis [20].

Pearls/Pitfalls

1. Take a good history. Helpful discussion topics with the patient that include acuity in onset, laterality, vision changes, pain with or without movement, trauma history, prior episodes, immune status such as HIV or steroid use, work environment, eye history including prior surgeries or contact use, and medication history can be helpful in differentiating the cause.
2. With chemical and burn injuries being an exception, a complete and thorough ocular examination should be performed prior to treatment. Remember, the visual acuity is the vital sign of the eye.
3. Remember that not all ocular pain is ocular in origin. It can be referred pain from the sinuses, dental in origin, or a manifestation of a neurological condition. Pay special attention to the neurological, musculoskeletal, and dermatological findings on examination when considering possible systemic disorders.
4. Emergent referral to an ophthalmologist is required for chemical and thermal burns, optic neuritis, herpes zoster ophthalmicus, corneal ulcers, and acute angle closure glaucoma.
5. Urgent referral or evaluation within 24–48 h is needed for keratitis, corneal abrasions, uveitis, scleritis, and episcleritis.

References

1. Alexander KL, Dull MW, Lalle PA, Magnus DE, Onofrey B. Care of the patient with anterior uveitis. In: Optometric clinical practice guideline. St. Louis: American Optometric Association; 1994. Revised 1994. Reviewed 2004.
2. Lachkar Y, Bouassida W. Drug-induced acute angle closure glaucoma. Curr Opin Ophthalmol. 2007;18(2):129–33.

3. Walker RA, Adhikari S. Chapter 241. Eye emergencies. In: Tintinalli JE, et al., editors. Tintinalli's emergency medicine: a comprehensive study guide, 8e. New York: McGraw-Hill; 2016. n. pag. AccessMedicine.

4. Dargin JM, Lowenstein RA. The painful eye. Emerg Med Clin North Am. 2008;26(1):199–216, viii.

5. Biswell R. Chapter 6. Cornea. In: Riordan-Eva P, Cunningham Jr ET, editors. Vaughan & Asbury's general ophthalmology, 18e. New York: McGraw-Hill; 2011. AccessMedicine.

6. Deibel JP, Cowling K. Ocular inflammation and infection. Emerg Med Clin North Am. 2013;31(2):387–97.

7. Spector J, Fernandez WG. Chemical, thermal, and biological ocular exposures. Emerg Med Clin North Am. 2008;26(1):125–36, vii.

8. Nijm LM, et al. Chapter 5. Conjunctiva & tears. In: Riordan-Eva P, Cunningham Jr ET, editors. Vaughan & Asbury's general ophthalmology, 18e. New York: McGraw-Hill; 2011. n. pag. AccessMedicine.

9. Scott CA, Catania LJ, Larkin KM, Melton R, Semes LP, Shovlin JP. Care of the patient with ocular surface disorders. In: Optometric clinical practice guideline. 2nd ed. St. Louis: American Optometric Association; 1995. Revised 2003, Reviewed 2010.

10. Morris D, Latham E. Ulcers in the eye. J Emerg Med. 2012;42(1):62–4.

11. Swaminathan A, Otterness K, Milne K, Rezaie S. The safety of topical anesthetics in the treatment of corneal abrasions: a review. J Emerg Med. 2015;49(5):810–5.

12. Puls HA, Cabrera D, Murad MH, Erwin PJ, Bellolio MF. Safety and effectiveness of topical anesthetics in corneal abrasions: systematic review and meta-analysis. J Emerg Med. 2015;49(5):816–24.

13. Ball IM, Seabrook J, Desai N, Allen L, Anderson S. Dilute proparacaine for the management of acute corneal injuries in the emergency department. CJEM. 2010;12(5):389–96.

14. Romaniuk VM. Ocular trauma and other catastrophes. Emerg Med Clin North Am. 2013;31(2):399–411.

15. Jackson J, Carr LW, Fisch BM III, Malinovsky VE, Talley DK. Care of the patient with primary angle closure glaucoma. In: Optometric clinical practice guideline. St. Louis: American Optometric Association; 1994. Revised 1998, Reviewed 2001.

16. Cunningham ET, et al. Chapter 7. Uveal tract & sclera. In: Riordan-Eva P, Cunningham Jr ET, editors. Vaughan & Asbury's general ophthalmology, 18e. New York: McGraw-Hill; 2011. AccessMedicine.

17. Mueller JB, Mcstay CM. Ocular infection and inflammation. Emerg Med Clin North Am. 2008;26(1):57–72, vi.

18. Pringle E, Graham EM. Chapter 15. Ocular disorders associated with systemic diseases. In: Riordan-Eva P, Cunningham Jr ET, editors. Vaughan & Asbury's general ophthalmology, 18e. New York: McGraw-Hill; 2011. n. pag. AccessMedicine.

19. Vortmann M, Schneider JI. Acute monocular visual loss. Emerg Med Clin North Am. 2008;26(1):73–96, vi.

20. Magauran B. Conditions requiring emergency ophthalmologic consultation. Emerg Med Clin North Am. 2008;26(1):233–8, viii.

21. Augsburger JJ, Corrêa ZM. Chapter 19. Ophthalmic trauma. In: Riordan-Eva P, Cunningham Jr ET, editors. Vaughan & Asbury's general ophthalmology, 18e. New York: McGraw-Hill; 2011. n. pag. AccessMedicine.

Chapter 8
Acute Vision Loss

Brit Long and Alex Koyfman

Brief Introduction

Acute vision loss has many etiologies with a large differential. These conditions can range from benign to permanent vision loss. Many of these diagnoses are time-sensitive, and the emergency physician may improve patient outcome through the consideration of several acute etiologies.

Clinical Presentation

Acute vision loss is defined by visual deficit lasting less than 24 h upon evaluation. Persistent visual loss is dysfunction lasting greater than 24 h [1–3]. Usually one eye is affected with reduction in vision to 20/200 or worse [1–3]. Several classification systems exist for acute vision loss. The usual classifica-

B. Long, MD (✉)
San Antonio Military Medical Center, Department of Emergency Medicine, San Antonio, TX, USA

A. Koyfman, MD
The University of Texas Southwestern Medical Center, Department of Emergency Medicine, Dallas, TX, USA

© Springer International Publishing AG, part of Springer Nature 2018
B. Long, A. Koyfman (eds.), *Handbook of Emergency Ophthalmology*, https://doi.org/10.1007/978-3-319-78945-3_8

135

tion scheme includes painful and painless vision loss, while a second utilizes anatomical location.

Differential Diagnosis

The differential of painful vision loss includes acute glaucoma, optic neuritis, giant cell arteritis (GCA), uveitis, and migraine headache. Painless causes include central retinal artery occlusion (CRAO), central retinal vein occlusion (CRVO), ischemic optic neuropathy, cataract, vitreous hemorrhage, amaurosis fugax, TIA, cortical blindness, retinal detachment, macular degeneration, diabetic retinopathy, CMV retinitis, methanol intoxication, and functional visual loss.

The other classification system relying on the visual pathway divides lesions into the media, retina, and neural pathways. Lesions affecting the media include keratopathy, vitreous hemorrhage, uveitis, endophthalmitis, hyphema, and lens pathology. Retina pathology includes retinal detachment, vascular occlusion, and acute maculopathy. Neural pathway lesions include those of the optic nerve, optic chiasm, and retrochiasm, including the posterior occipital lobe.

Other important factors include relative afferent pupillary defect, speed of onset, fundoscopic examination, ultrasound findings, and specific history and physical examination findings.

Clinical Evaluation

History

Several aspects of the history are important. First, a distinction should be made on whether the visual loss was acute or if preexisting visual deficit was present before the onset of worsening vision loss [1–3].

- Determine whether the visual deficit occurs in one eye or both eyes.
- Determine the quality and area of visual loss (is it both sides and one particular area of visual loss).

- Ask about pain. Acute glaucoma may present with deep, boring pain and nausea/vomiting, while endophthalmitis also presents with boring pain. Optic neuritis is associated with increased pain with eye movement.
- Evaluate for redness and discharge.
- Determine whether trauma was involved. Uveitis/iritis can cause decreased vision, as can ruptured globe, hyphema, traumatic cataract, or retinal detachment.
- Evaluate for other symptoms such as neurologic deficit (including weakness accompanying a stroke).

The *past medical history* including vascular disease (diabetes, hypertension, hypercoagulability, etc.), refractive status (near-sighted individuals are at higher risk for retinal tears and detachment), use of contact lens (risk for keratitis, abrasion, ulcer), history of eye surgery (increased patient risk for uveitis, iritis, glaucoma, retinal detachment, and infection), and finally medications (which often have visual side effects) [1–3].

1. Medications affecting vision include anticholinergics (accommodation loss, glaucoma), bisphosphonates (uveitis), digoxin (yellow-tinged vision), rifabutin (uveitis), sildenafil (blue-tinged vision, ischemic neuropathy), sulfa agents (myopia), topiramate (glaucoma), OCPs (ischemic events), and cancer medications.

Physical Examination

After the focused history, a complete physical exam can provide a great deal of vital information. Many emergency physicians are uncomfortable completing ophthalmologic exams, but this is an essential aspect of the care we provide. The following should be assessed in the patient with visual loss [1–3].

1. *General inspection*: evaluate the lids and sclera closely for erythema, tearing, light sensitivity, proptosis, and ptosis.
2. *Visual acuity*: this can often be done before the patient is roomed for provider evaluation. Acuity should be completed with correction based on a Snellen eye chart, each eye separately and then together.

    (a) If the patient does not have glasses in his/her position, a pinhole can be used to assist with correction.

    (b) If unable to see the letters, ability to detect hand motion, movement, or light should be assessed.

3. *Pupils* for symmetry, light reactivity, and pupillary reflex.
4. *Extraocular movements* including cranial nerves III, IV, and VI.
5. *Confrontation* visual fields.
6. Apply *fluorescein* and evaluate for abrasion, ulcer, and Seidel's sign.
7. Evaluate *intraocular pressure* by tonometry. Normal values are 10–20 mm Hg.
8. *Slit lamp* evaluating the anterior (and posterior chambers, though dilated exam with fundoscopy is needed to definitely evaluate posterior chambers) is important for visualization of cell and flare.
9. *Ocular US* is a high yield test for emergency physicians. The anterior chamber, lens, posterior chamber/retina, and optic nerve can be evaluated using US, making this essential in ocular evaluation.

Clinical Conditions and Management

Media Problems

(a) *Open globe* is one ophthalmologic condition that requires immediate treatment. Any trauma including paintball or BB guns can cause open globe, and the majority of patients are male. This injury is normally apparent on exam, which reveals laceration, volume loss of eye, uveal prolapse, peaked/eccentric pupil, 360° subconjunctival hemorrhage, or a foreign body. Visual acuity is often significantly decreased (Fig. 8.1). Ophthalmology should be immediately consulted, and CT scan is often required for foreign body evaluation. Treatment requires keeping the patient NPO, avoiding FB removal, avoiding eye manipulation, eye shield placement, head of bed elevation to at

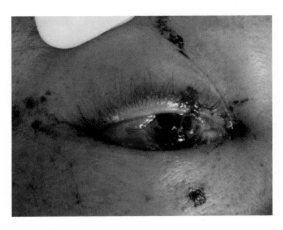

FIGURE 8.1 Shotgun injury to the right eye with hyphema (iris details are obscured), soft globe, and bullous subconjunctival hemorrhage (Image from http://webeye.ophth.uiowa.edu/eyeforum/tutorials/trauma.htm. The author(s)/editor(s) and publishers acknowledge the University of Iowa and EyeRounds.org for permission to reproduce this copyrighted material)

least 30°, aggressive nausea treatment, analgesia, and IV antibiotics including vancomycin plus fluoroquinolone or ceftazidime. Urgent surgical repair within 24 h of injury is associated with the best outcomes [1–6].

(b) *Conjunctivitis* is rarely a cause of vision loss, except in the case of chlamydia trachomatis. On the other hand, keratitis can contribute to vision loss. Infectious causes include bacteria, herpes simplex, and adenovirus [1–3, 7, 8].

(c) *Hyphema* is a collection of blood in the anterior chamber, most commonly resulting from blunt trauma (Fig. 8.2). Hyphema size is related to outcome. Vision loss occurs in the setting of large hyphema (as the visual axis is obstructed), as well as the development of rebleeding or acute glaucoma. Evaluate for other signs of trauma, including other ophthalmologic trauma. Emergent ophthalmology consultation is needed in the setting of marked decreased VA, signs of open globe, and large cir-

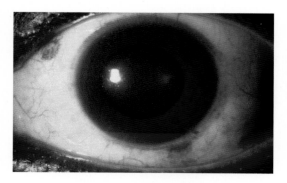

FIGURE 8.2 Traumatic hyphema with RBC layering (Image from http://webeye.ophth.uiowa.edu/eyeforum/atlas/pages/Hyphema/index.htm. The author(s)/editor(s) and publishers acknowledge the University of Iowa and EyeRounds.org for permission to reproduce this copyrighted material)

cumferential hemorrhage. Same-day evaluation is recommended for patients with hyphema and intense eye pain, grossly visible blood in the anterior chamber, or damage to adjacent structures. In the setting of significant hyphema, labs (CBC, coagulation panel, sickle cell testing) and CT should be completed. Treatment is similar to patients with open globe. Nausea should be treated, and pain controlled with topical pain treatment including cycloplegics if open globe has been excluded [1–3, 9–12].

(d) *Iritis* often results in pain, photophobia, and vision loss in the extreme form. This is often deep, aching pain that radiates to the temporal regions. Trauma, infection, and rheumatologic conditions may result in iritis. Exam will reveal ciliary flush (erythema closer to the iris as opposed to the periphery), consensual photophobia, and slit lamp with cells and flare with hypopyon. Treatment requires cycloplegics (homatropine 1 drop TID, cyclopentolate 1 drop TID) and ophthalmology evaluation. Steroids can be used but only in association with ophthalmologist consultation [1–3, 13–15].

(e) *Glaucoma*, particularly acute angle closure, often presents with acute painful vision loss. Nausea/vomiting, blurry

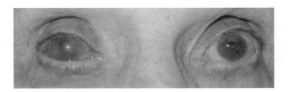

FIGURE 8.3 Acute angle closure glaucoma with hazy cornea and mid-dilated pupil (Image from https://webeye.ophth.uiowa.edu/eyeforum/atlas/pages/acute-angle-closure.html. The author(s)/editor(s) and publishers acknowledge the University of Iowa and EyeRounds.org for permission to reproduce this copyrighted material)

vision with halos around lights, and photophobia are other common symptoms. Diagnosis requires intraocular pressure >21 mm Hg (usually greater than 40 mm Hg), though conjunctival injection, corneal edema with hazy/fixed/dilated pupil, and shallow anterior chamber (Fig. 8.3) are common. Risk factors include far-sighted patients, transition from light to dark environments, and dilating medications. Management requires immediate ophthalmologic consultation, followed by medications including topical beta-blocker (timolol 0.25–0.5%), topical cholinergic agent (pilocarpine 1 drop) after timolol, and parenteral acetazolamide 500 mg IV with mannitol 1.25–2 g/kg IV if required [1–3, 16, 17].

(f) *Vitreous hemorrhage* often occurs with trauma, though spontaneous vitreous detachment and retinal tear can also result in this condition. The amount of blood contained in the vitreous is proportional to the amount of vision loss. Symptoms include floaters, reddish tint to vision, and brief flashes of light seen by the patient in peripheral vision fields (known as photopsia). Decreased red reflex is often seen on exam, and the retina may not be visible on fundoscopy due to the presence of blood. US will reveal horizontal, minimally echogenic structures behind the lens. Treatment includes ensuring patient head elevation to 30–45° and ophthalmologic consultation for definitive treatment. Anticoagulation should be avoided. It often takes months to completely clear the hemorrhage [1–3, 18, 19].

Of note, it is often difficult to differentiate on US vitreous hemorrhage and retinal detachment. However, there are three distinct findings that will help distinguish the two: retinal detachments can be followed posteriorly to the optic disk, vitreous hemorrhages remain horizontal when the patient moves the eye side to side, and vitreous hemorrhages are often seen in the middle section of the posterior eye.

(g) *Posterior vitreous detachment* (PVD) is common in patients over 60 years and occurs with vitreous gel pulling away from the retina. Patients with nearsightedness (myopia) are at greater risk, similar to retinal detachment. This can also occur after cataract surgery. Symptoms include flashes of light and floaters. This may lead to retinal detachment, with greatest risk within the first 6 weeks of symptom onset. These patients require ophthalmology consultation [1–3, 19].

(h) *Endophthalmitis* refers to infection in the eye, particularly of the vitreous and aqueous humor. This is usually due to inoculation of organisms through trauma, surgery, or keratitis. Bacteria are most common, but fungal and viral causes can also cause this. Symptoms progress quickly over 12–24 h including decreased vision and dull eye pain, though patients commonly display no signs of sepsis (SIRS negative). The lids are often normal, but the conjunctiva will be injected and edematous (Fig. 8.4). Decreased VA with hypopyon is often found with haziness of the retinal view. Cells and flare will be seen on slit lamp. US may demonstrate increased echogenicity within the vitreous material. This disease is a medical emergency requiring ophthalmologic evaluation for vitrectomy and antibiotics (vancomycin and ceftazidime) injected into the vitreous material. Intravenous antibiotics can be provided, but they will not be effective in clearing infection [1–3, 16, 20].

(i) *Lens pathology* can affect vision. Any change in the size, clarity, or positioning of the lens changes the focus of light on the retina, which results in vision changes. Trauma

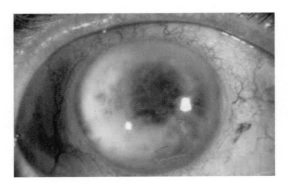

FIGURE 8.4 Endophthalmitis with hazy cornea and hypopyon (Image from http://www.eyerounds.org/atlas/pages/endophthalmitis-sp/ Fungal-Endo-LRG.jpg. The author(s)/editor(s) and publishers acknowledge the University of Iowa and EyeRounds.org for permission to reproduce this copyrighted material)

causing lens dislocation is the most common cause of sudden vision loss due to lens pathology. Chronic cataracts will cause gradual vision loss [1–3].

Retina

(a) *Retinal detachment* can occur in the setting of trauma but is often not associated with an instigating event. Three mechanisms exist: rhegmatogenous (most common), exudative, and tractional. Sudden onset of new floaters, black dots, and flashes of light are common symptoms. Early stages may present with visual field loss, but if the macula or central retina becomes involved, visual acuity is severely affected. This is not painful. Afferent pupillary defect may be present, but no signs of red eye will be present. US will be the key to diagnosis, which will demonstrate a highly reflective, mobile undulating membrane (Fig. 8.5). Treatment requires emergent ophthalmology consultation and evaluation [1–3, 16, 18, 21].

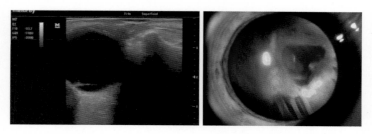

FIGURE 8.5 US (left) and slit lamp (right) of retinal detachment (Images from https://vimeo.com/127186824 and https://upload.wikimedia.org/wikipedia/commons/b/b0/Slit_lamp_photograph_showing_retinal_detachment_in_Von_Hippel-Lindau_disease_EDA08.JPG)

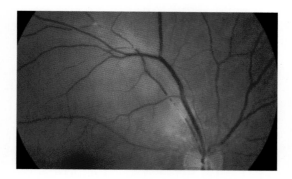

FIGURE 8.6 Fundoscopic exam revealing CRAO (Image from http://webeye.ophth.uiowa.edu/eyeforum/atlas/pages/BRAO-Branched-Retinal-Artery-Occlusion.html. The author(s)/editor(s) and publishers acknowledge the University of Iowa and EyeRounds.org for permission to reproduce this copyrighted material)

(b) *Vascular occlusion* consists of central retinal artery occlusion (CRAO) and central retinal vein occlusion (CRVO). CRAO presents with sudden, painless, severe vision loss, usually monocular and central (Fig. 8.6). VA is seriously affected. This disease usually affects elderly patients with carotid vascular disease, though pediatric patients with blood disorders including leukemia or

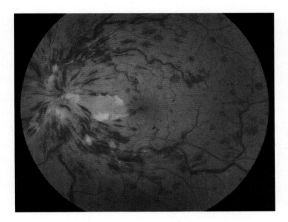

FIGURE 8.7 Fundoscopic exam revealing CRVO (Image from http://webeye.ophth.uiowa.edu/eyeforum/atlas/pages/CRVO-w-CLRAO/CRVO-CLRAO-LRG.jpg. The author(s)/editor(s) and publishers acknowledge the University of Iowa and EyeRounds.org for permission to reproduce this copyrighted material)

sickle cell disease can experience this. A pale retina with cherry red macula is seen on fundoscopic exam. Evaluation with ECG, CBC, coag panel, echocardiogram (for emboli), and carotid US is needed. Ophthalmology emergent evaluation is required. Ocular massage with intermittent pressure applied, timolol ophthalmic drops, increase PCO_2 (rebreathing or carbogen), and acetazolamide IV are standard ED treatments, but ophthalmology consultation is required [1–3, 16, 22, 23]. *CRVO* is due to thrombosis of the central retinal vein with disc swelling, preretinal hemorrhage, and cotton wool spots with the classic "blood and thunder" appearance (Fig. 8.7). The onset is typically subacute as opposed to the sudden onset vision loss of CRAO. A relative pupillary defect is common. Risk factors include HTN, DM, vasculitis, and glaucoma. Diagnosis is with fundoscopy. Ophthalmology should be consulted, but unfortunately no treatment regimen provides consistent results.

Possible treatments include aspirin, anticoagulation, photocoagulation, and intravitreal injections [1–3, 16, 23, 24].

(c) *Acute maculopathy* often results in central field vision loss with distortion in other fields. This is usually common and progressive, as opposed to sudden onset. Macula pathology including macular degeneration and diabetic retinopathy are the usual causes. Diagnosis requires dilated ophthalmologic examination.

(d) *Giant cell arteritis* or *temporal arteritis* can be a cause of CRAO or ischemic optic neuropathy. This disease is predominantly seen in older patients over 50 years. Women and Caucasians are the classic patient population, and the presentation usually entails headache (temporal location), jaw claudication, fever, weight loss, general fatigue, and tenderness to palpation along the temporal artery with decreased pulsation. Jaw claudication and diplopia are the most predictive symptoms, with prominent/tender temporal artery the most predictive sign. Elevated ESR and CRP can help suggest diagnosis, but normal values should not rule this out. Definitive diagnosis requires biopsy of the temporal artery. Treatment should be started with high-dose methylprednisolone 1 g IV in those with vision changes. Vision loss unfortunately is usually complete and irreversible [1–3, 25–27].

Neural Pathway

(a) *Optic neuritis* is due to inflammation, demyelination, or degeneration of the optic nerve. It is most commonly seen in females ages 15–45 years. This disease is usually monocular and causes severe eye pain with brief flashes of light. The patient often experiences severe photophobia and decreased red vision or dyschromatopsia. In children, this may follow bacterial or viral infections, as well as Lyme disease. This can also be a presenting sign of multiple sclerosis, especially in adults. Exam will reveal marked VA decrease with afferent pupillary defect. Otherwise, the exam is often normal. Treatment requires IV steroids with methyl-prednisolone 250 mg IV TID, followed by PO steroids. Further workup requires ophthalmologic consultation and MRI of the head to evaluate for white matter plaque presence [1–3, 28–31].

(b) *Orbital infection*, particularly orbital cellulitis, leads to visual loss in the later stages of disease. This disease of the posterior orbital septum begins in the sinuses most commonly. Clinical signs/symptoms of orbital cellulitis are fever, proptosis, down and out globe position, limited and often painful eye movements, double vision, and later vision loss. Physical examination will reveal the diagnosis, though CT of the orbit is often needed for prognostication and to evaluate the extent of the infection. This disease can rapidly progress intracranially to form abscesses, meningitis, or cavernous sinus thrombosis. Treatment requires admission, IV antibiotics, and ophthalmology/ENT consultation [1–3, 32–35].

(c) *Cavernous sinus thrombosis* may lead to visual loss through thrombosis of ophthalmic vasculature or compression of the optic nerve. This disease often begins with infection in the sinuses. Diagnosis requires MRI/MRV or CTA/venography. Antibiotics with anticoagulation are often needed [1–3, 36, 37].

(d) *Idiopathic intracranial hypertension* is due to increased ICP with compression of the optic nerve. No space-occupying lesion or infection is present in this disease. Obesity and medications (steroids, tetracycline, vitamin A, ddAVP) are associated with development of this disease. Patients often have headache, transient visual defects, and papilledema. Diagnosis requires imaging with lumbar puncture, which demonstrates elevated pressures. Complete vision loss may occur and starts with transient visual loss [1–3, 38, 39].

(e) *Optic nerve ischemia* and nerve avulsion in the setting of trauma may cause blindness. Occipital lobe lesions in the setting of ischemic or hemorrhagic infarction can lead to vision loss acutely as well. This would be due to ischemia in the posterior circulation of the cerebral vasculature [1–3, 16, 40].

(f) *Optic pathway tumors* such as glioma may present with sudden visual loss, but usually visual deficits are progressive over time. The optic chiasm may also be affected, causing bitemporal hemianopia [1–3, 41].

Ingestions

(a) Several toxins can lead to blindness. Thus, this must be considered in the ED evaluation of sudden visual loss, especially bilateral. This is often not at the forefront on the ED differential. Methanol overdose causes direct optic nerve toxicity from formate production and can occur up to 72 h after ingestion. Symptoms often begin with blind spots, decreased color vision, and blurriness. Eye exam may reveal mydriasis, retinal edema, and hyperemia of the optic disk. Afferent pupillary defect is a late and poor prognostic finding. Treatment includes fomepizole and ophthalmology consultation [1–3, 42, 43].

(b) Other toxins or medications leading to cerebral ischemia or hypoxia can contribute to cortical blindness. Optic ischemia with carbon monoxide, direct neurotoxicity from cisplatin, local vasospasm from amphetamines or cocaine, and shock from antihypertensive agents (beta and calcium blockers) are associated with blindness. Other toxins affecting vision include barbiturates, chloramphenicol, emetine, ethambutol, isoniazid, and heavy metals [1–3].

Functional Vision Loss

Functional vision loss is a diagnosis of exclusion and not a diagnosis for the ED. This is defined as vision loss without organic pathology or disease. Purposeful feigning of blindness occurs with malingering, while patients with conversion disorder perceive true blindness but lack concern for their symptoms. The exam of the eye will be normal. Nystagmus with optokinetic drug can prove vision presence. A second way of evaluating vision is placing a mirror in front of the patient and having the patient open his/her eyes. If the patient tracks the mirror, vision loss is not present [1–3].

Disposition

The emergency physician plays a key role in the assessment and management of acute vision loss. Immediate treatment is needed for acute central retinal artery occlusion, acute glaucoma, and giant cell arteritis. Emergent referral to ophthalmology is required for open globe, chemical burn, endophthalmitis, hyphema, retinal detachment, and infectious keratitis. Urgent referral, or evaluation within 24–48 h, is needed for uveitis, vitreous hemorrhage, acute maculopathy, central retinal vein occlusion, and optic neuritis [1–3].

Pearls and Pitfalls

Ophthalmologic complaints involving sudden vision loss are something many physicians shy away from. However, these conditions can cause significant patient morbidity.

1. History including specific eye involvement, sudden vs. chronic loss, pain, redness and discharge, trauma, other symptoms, and medication use are vital.
2. Physicians should be comfortable completing an appropriate history and physical examination including general inspection, visual acuity, pupils, EOMs, visual fields, fluorescein, lids, IOP, slit lamp, and US.
3. Emergent consultation is required for acute angle closure glaucoma, retinal detachment, CRAO, open globe, endophthalmitis, chemical burn, infectious keratitis, and giant cell arteritis.

4. Urgent referral is needed for uveitis, vitreous hemorrhage, acute maculopathy, CRVO, and optic neuritis.
5. Keep in mind other etiologies of vision loss including ischemia, stroke, toxin, infection, and functional.

References

1. Burde R, Savino P, Trobe J. Clinical decisions in neuro-ophthalmology. 3rd ed. St. Louis: Mosby; 2002.
2. Walker RA, Adhikaris S. Chap. 241. Eye emergencies. In: Tintinalli's emergency medicine: a comprehensive study guide. 8th ed. New York: McGraw-Hill; 2016.
3. Guluma K, Lee JE. Ophthalmology. In: Rosen's emergency medicine, Chapter 61. p. 780–8190.e3.
4. Colby K. Management of open globe injuries. Int Ophthalmol Clin. 1999;39:59.
5. Unver YB, Kapran Z, Acar N, Altan T. Ocular trauma score in open-globe injuries. J Trauma. 2009;66:1030.
6. Thakker MM, Ray S. Vision-limiting complications in open-globe injuries. Can J Ophthalmol. 2006;41:86.
7. Friedlaender MH. A review of the causes and treatment of bacterial and allergic conjunctivitis. Clin Ther. 1995;17:800.
8. Weiss A, Brinser JH, Nazar-Stewart V. Acute conjunctivitis in childhood. J Pediatr. 1993;122:10.
9. Walton W, Von Hagen S, Grigorian R, Zarbin M. Management of traumatic hyphema. Surv Ophthalmol. 2002;47:297.
10. Brandt MT, Haug RH. Traumatic hyphema: a comprehensive review. J Oral Maxillofac Surg. 2001;59:1462.
11. Pashby T. Eye injuries in Canadian amateur hockey. Can J Ophthalmol. 1985;20:2.
12. Sankar PS, Chen TC, Grosskreutz CL, Pasquale LR. Traumatic hyphema. Int Ophthalmol Clin. 2002;42:57.
13. Guly CM, Forrester JV. Investigation and management of uveitis. BMJ. 2010;341:c4976.
14. Jabs DA, Busingye J. Approach to the diagnosis of the uveitides. Am J Ophthalmol. 2013;156:228.
15. Rosenbaum JT. Nibbling away at the diagnosis of idiopathic uveitis. JAMA Ophthalmol. 2015;133:146.
16. Pokhrel PK, Loftus SA. Ocular emergencies. Am Fam Physician. 2007;76:829.

17. See JLS, PTK C. Angle-closure glaucoma. In: Yanoff M, Duker JS, editors. Ophthalmology. 3rd ed. St. Louis: Mosby; 2009. p. 1162.

18. D'Amico DJ. Clinical practice. Primary retinal detachment. N Engl J Med. 2008;359:2346.

19. Hikichi T, Trempe CL, Schepens CL. Posterior vitreous detachment as a risk factor for retinal detachment. Ophthalmology. 1995;102:527.

20. Mandelbaum S, Forster RK. Exogenous endophthalmitis. In: Pepose JS, Holland GN, Wilhelmus KR, editors. Ocular immunology and infection. St. Louis: Mosby; 1996. p. 1298.

21. Eagle RC Jr. Mechanisms of maculopathy. Ophthalmology. 1984;91:613.

22. Appen RE, Wray SH, Cogan DG. Central retinal artery occlusion. Am J Ophthalmol. 1975;79:374.

23. Hayreh SS, Podhajsky PA, Zimmerman MB. Natural history of visual outcome in central retinal vein occlusion. Ophthalmology. 2011;118:119.

24. Eye Disease Case-Control Study Group. Risk factors for central retinal vein occlusion. Arch Ophthalmol. 1996;114:545.

25. Smetana GW, Shmerling RH. Does this patient have temporal arteritis? JAMA. 2002;287:92.

26. Younge BR, Cook BE Jr, Bartley GB, et al. Initiation of glucocorticoid therapy: before or after temporal artery biopsy? Mayo Clin Proc. 2004;79:483.

27. Hunder GG. Giant cell arteritis and polymyalgia rheumatica. In: Kelly WN, Harris ED, Ruddy S, Sledge CB, editors. Textbook of Rheumatology. 5th ed. Philadelphia: WB Saunders; 1996.

28. Balcer LJ. Clinical practice. Optic neuritis. N Engl J Med. 2006;354:1273.

29. Foroozan R, Buono LM, Savino PJ, Sergott RC. Acute demyelinating optic neuritis. Curr Opin Ophthalmol. 2002;13:375.

30. Frohman EM, Frohman TC, Zee DS, et al. The neuroophthalmology of multiple sclerosis. Lancet Neurol. 2005;4:111.

31. Arnold AC. Evolving management of optic neuritis and multiple sclerosis. Am J Ophthalmol. 2005;139:1101.

32. Seltz LB, Smith J, Durairaj VD, et al. Microbiology and antibiotic management of orbital cellulitis. Pediatrics. 2011;127:e566.

33. Nageswaran S, Woods CR, Benjamin DK Jr, et al. Orbital cellulitis in children. Pediatr Infect Dis J. 2006;25:695.

34. Zhang J, Stringer MD. Ophthalmic and facial veins are not valveless. Clin Exp Ophthalmol. 2010;38:502.

35. Mills R. Orbital and periorbital sepsis. J Laryngol Otol. 1987;101:1242.
36. Ferro JM, Canhão P, Stam J, et al. Prognosis of cerebral vein and dural sinus thrombosis: results of the International Study on Cerebral Vein and Dural Sinus Thrombosis (ISCVT). Stroke. 2004;35:664.
37. Saposnik G, Barinagarrementeria F, Brown RD Jr, et al. Diagnosis and management of cerebral venous thrombosis: a statement for healthcare professionals from the American Heart Association/American Stroke Association. Stroke. 2011;42:1158.
38. Acheson JF. Idiopathic intracranial hypertension and visual function. Br Med Bull. 2006;79–80:233.
39. Wall M, Kupersmith MJ, Kieburtz KD, et al. The idiopathic intracranial hypertension treatment trial: clinical profile at baseline. JAMA Neurol. 2014;71:693.
40. Rucker JC, Biousse V, Newman NJ. Ischemic optic neuropathies. Curr Opin Neurol. 2004;17:27.
41. Alvord EC Jr, Lofton S. Gliomas of the optic nerve or chiasm. Outcome by patients' age, tumor site, and treatment. J Neurosurg. 1988;68:85.
42. Barceloux DG, Bond GR, Krenzelok EP, et al. American Academy of Clinical Toxicology practice guidelines on the treatment of methanol poisoning. J Toxicol Clin Toxicol. 2002;40:415.
43. Sivilotti ML. Methanol intoxication. Ann Emerg Med. 2000;35:313.

Chapter 9
Acute Angle-Closure Glaucoma

Dustin Williams

Clinical Presentation

Acute angle-closure glaucoma is a major cause of vision loss and is an optic neuropathy caused by an acute increase in intraocular pressures due to obstructed outflow of aqueous humor from the anterior chamber of the eye [1–5]. Aqueous humor is made by the ciliary process in the posterior chamber and is circulated to the anterior chamber through the pupil. In a healthy eye, the aqueous humor then drains through the trabecular meshwork into the canal of Schlemm. However, in acute angle-closure glaucoma, this normal flow is interrupted due to a narrowing of the anterior chamber angle causing an occlusion of the trabecular meshwork [1–9].

Acute angle-closure glaucoma can be categorized into primary angle closure and secondary angle closure. Primary angle closure is caused by anatomic variants that predispose some people to have an obstruction of the anterior chamber angle. This is contrasted to secondary acute angle-closure glaucoma that causes obstruction secondary to an associated event or insult. Primary acute angle-closure glaucoma is usu-

D. Williams, MD
UT Southwestern Medical Center, Dallas, TX, USA
e-mail: dustin.williams@utsouthwestern.edu

© Springer International Publishing AG, part of Springer Nature 2018
B. Long, A. Koyfman (eds.), *Handbook of Emergency Ophthalmology*, https://doi.org/10.1007/978-3-319-78945-3_9

153

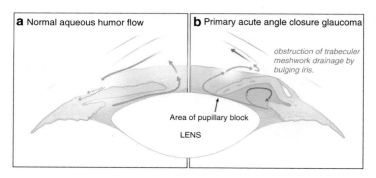

FIGURE 9.1 Circulation of aqueous humor in normal eye compared with pupillary block in primary acute angle-closure glaucoma

ally secondary to a pupil block by which the posterior iris becomes affixed to the lens which results in increased pressure in the posterior chamber. This results in a forward bowing of the peripheral iris that then results in an appositional closure of the anterior chamber angle, and thus, trabecular meshwork drainage of aqueous humor decrease, increasing intraocular pressure (Fig. 9.1) [1, 3–7].

Patients usually present with abrupt onset monocular pain with severe visual impairment and red eye; however, they may present with more nonspecific complaints of headache, nausea, and vomiting. The speed of onset and magnitude of elevation of intraocular pressure determines the severity of patient symptoms [1, 3–7, 10, 11]. Clinicians should perform a detailed ocular examination in any patient presenting with a headache as acute angle-closure glaucoma is often missed when patients present with primarily systemic symptoms rather than ocular symptoms [9, 12]. This acute angle closure is often triggered by pupil dilation, such as dim illumination, accommodation, sympathetic arousal, and medications. Patients may report a recent history of intermittent eye pain as acute angle-closure glaucoma crisis can be self-limiting, resolve spontaneously, and may reoccur.

Risk Factors

Risk factors for acute angle-closure glaucoma can be described in terms of demographic or ocular features. Demographic features include a family history of angle closure, older age (thicker lens), Asian or Inuit ethnicity, and female gender. In terms of ocular risk factors, acute angle-closure glaucoma is predisposed in those patients with shallow anterior chambers, hyperopia (farsightedness), and short axial length of the eye, which places patients at a higher risk for "pupillary block" due to a crowded anterior chamber [1, 4–7, 13]. Many medications are also associated with inducing acute angle closure secondary to pupillary dilation (Table 9.1) [1].

TABLE 9.1 Medications associated with acute angle closure [1]	
Psychiatric medications	
Selective serotonin reuptake inhibitors	
Tricyclic antidepressants	
Sympathomimetic	
Amphetamine, cocaine	
Anticholinergics	
Eye drops (mydriatics)	
Inhaled (ipratropium)	
Systemic (atropine, scopolamine patches)	
Anticonvulsants	
Topiramate	
Diuretics	
Hydrochlorothiazide	

Evaluation (Exam and History Findings)

Most patients with acute angle-closure crisis present with complaints of monocular eye pain and severe visual impairments, often reporting halos around lights. Patients may present with more nonspecific complaints of associated nausea with vomiting and headache. A comprehensive ocular exam is imperative in any patient that one suspects acute angle closure, including visual acuity, intraocular pressures, slit lamp exam of anterior segment, and visual field testing [12]. Clinicians should also take a detailed history for medications that could contribute to angle closure, and patients should also be asked about a history of, or family history of, angle closure.

In acute angle-closure crisis, an acute increase in intraocular pressure causes marked vascular congestion of conjunctival and episcleral vessels with a cloudy, hazy cornea secondary to increased intraocular pressures overwhelming the corneal endothelial pumps, allowing water to enter the cornea (Fig. 9.2). Clinicians may also see a sluggish to fixed midposition to dilated pupil (secondary to pupillary block) with very high intraocular pressures, usually greater than 30 mmHg.

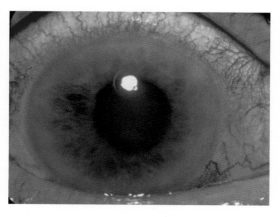

FIGURE 9.2 Acute angle-closure glaucoma. Licensed under the Creative Commons

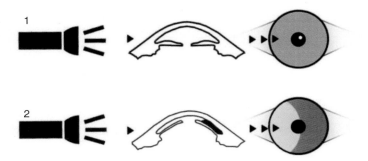

FIGURE 9.3 Oblique flashlight test in normal eye (1) and in acute angle closure (2)

Pressures may reach 60–80 mmHg. Crisis can be exacerbated by dim environments, reading small print, and emotional upset. In addition to any other causes of pupillary dilation, this mild dilation allows for maximal pupil block, and then the mild peripheral iris laxity balloons forward, obstructing the anterior chamber angle [3–7].

Clinicians should be able to estimate the anterior chamber depth with the oblique flashlight test, in which the clinician holds a flashlight on the temporal aspect of the eye and provides tangential light across the anterior chamber, parallel to the iris. If a shadow appears along the nasal aspect of the iris, the anterior chamber angle is narrow. The shallow anterior chamber can be confirmed with slit lamp exam of the anterior chamber (Fig. 9.3) [7].

Applanation tonometry should be performed to approximate intraocular pressure and can be greater than 60–80 mmHg. If patients have markedly elevated pressures, they may present with a firm, rock hard, and tender globe.

Management/Treatment

Acute angle-closure glaucoma requires prompt diagnosis and treatment to preserve vision. The definitive treatment requires laser peripheral iridotomy, in which a laser is used

TABLE 9.2 Medical treatment of acute angle-closure glaucoma [1]

Treatment	Medication	Method	Notes
Beta-blockers	Timolol 0.5%	Decrease aqueous production	Caution in asthma/COPD
Carbonic anhydrate inhibitors	Acetazolamide 500 mg PO Acetazolamide 500 mg IV	Decrease aqueous production	Caution in patients with sulfa allergy
α_2 Adrenergic agonist	Brimonidine 0.15%	Decrease aqueous production/ increase aqueous outflow	Can have acute reduction in aqueous outflow but increased outflow with prolonged use
Prostaglandin analog	Latanoprost 0.005%	Increase aqueous outflow	
Cholinergics	Pilocarpine 1–2%	Increase aqueous outflow	Not effective at high IOP
Steroids (topical)	Prednisolone 1%	Decrease inflammation	Use in consultation with ophthalmology
Hyperosmotic agents	Mannitol 1–2 g/kg IV	Decrease vitreous volume	

to create an artificial opening in the iris to release the "pupillary block" (which will also need to be performed on the fellow eye to prevent any possibility of acute angle closure in that eye) [6, 9, 11, 12]. The keystone of treatment in the emergency department is medical management to acutely lower intraocular pressure. This is accomplished via multiple modalities which typically utilize a combination of carbonic anhydrase inhibitors, beta-blockers, miotics, and hyperosmotics which serve to (1) decrease production of aqueous humor, (2) increase outflow of aqueous humor, or (3) decrease volume of vitreous humor (Table 9.2) [3–5, 14, 15].

Intraocular pressure should be checked 30–60 min after initiation of medical treatment in order to ensure improving intraocular pressure. These patients require a comprehensive eye examination and prompt ophthalmological consultation [1, 9]. Often times, iridotomy is delayed secondary to corneal edema, and medical therapy is initiated to lower the intraocular pressure acutely; however, iridotomy should be performed as soon as possible. Analgesics and antiemetics should also be used symptomatically in these patients [1, 14].

Pearls/Pitfalls

Acute angle-closure glaucoma can present with a myriad of complaints and symptoms, requiring an astute clinician with a high index of suspicion.

1. Consider acute angle-closure glaucoma in patients presenting with headache, nausea/vomiting, and/or vision change.
2. Do not use dilating drops in acute angle glaucoma, as this could worsen outflow obstruction.
3. Use caution with topical beta-blockers in patients with reactive airway disease/asthma.
4. Acetazolamide is contraindicated in sulfa allergic patients.
5. Document an ocular exam in all patients presenting for headache and nausea/vomiting.
6. Usually unilateral but may present bilaterally, particularly when associated with a medication.
7. Patients will need definitive iridotomy and, usually, an iridotomy of the fellow eye.

References

1. Weizer J. Angle-closure glaucoma. In: UpToDate, Post TW, editor, Waltham, MA: UpToDate. Accessed 5 Aug 2016.
2. Tarongoy P, Lin C, Walton D. Angle-closure glaucoma: the role of the lens in the pathogenesis, prevention, and treatment. Surv Ophthalmol. 2009;54(2):211–25.
3. Walker RA, Adhikari S. Eye Emergencies. In: Tintinalli's emergency medicine: a comprehensive study guide. 7th ed. New York: McGraw Hill; 2015. Chap. 236.
4. Brunette DD. Ophthalmology. In: Rosen's emergency medicine. 7th ed. Philadelphia, PA: Elsevier/Saunders; 2017. p. 1055–6. Chap. 70.
5. Ehlers JP, Chirag PS. The wills eye manual: office and emergency room diagnosis and treatment of eye disease. Philadelphia, PA: Lippincott Williams & Wilkins; 2008.
6. Weinreb R, Aung T, Medeiros F. The pathophysiology and treatment of glaucoma: a review. JAMA. 2014;311(18):1901–11. https://doi.org/10.1001/jama.2014.3192.
7. Coleman AL. Glaucoma. Lancet. 1999;354(9192):1803–10.
8. Mahmood AR, Narang AT. Diagnosis and management of the acute red eye. Emerg Med Clin North Am. 2008;26:35–55.
9. Dargin JM, Lowenstein R. The painful eye. Emerg Med Clin North Am. 2008;26:199–216.
10. Berfkoff D, Sanchez L. An uncommon presentation of acute angle-closure glaucoma. J Emerg Med. 2005;29(1):43–4.
11. Ohringer G. Unilateral headache and loss of vision. BMJ. 2014;348:g1188.
12. Prum BE, et al. Primary angle closure preferred practice pattern® guidelines. Ophthalmology. 2016;123(1):P1–P40.
13. Patel K, Patel S. Angle-closure glaucoma. Dis Mon. 2014;60:254–62.
14. Choong YF, Irfan S, Menage M. Acute angle closure glaucoma: an evaluation of a protocol for acute treatment. Eye. 1999;13:613–6.
15. Emanuel ME, et al. Evidence-based management of primary angle closure glaucoma. Curr Opin Ophthalmol. 2014;25:89–92.

Chapter 10
Eye Infections

Matthew Streitz

Brief Introduction

Eye complaints account for approximately 1–2% of all ED visits [1, 2]. Eye emergencies can be categorized into three categories: the red eye, the painful eye, and those with associated vision loss. This chapter will focus mainly on eye infections and the most common disorders emergency department physicians need to be suspicious of, diagnose, and rapidly treat upon their presentation. This chapter will discuss the presentation, workup, treatment, and disposition for:

1. Periorbital cellulitis
2. Orbital cellulitis
3. Bacterial conjunctivitis
4. Viral conjunctivitis
5. Neonatal conjunctivitis
6. Contact lens complications (as they pertain to infectious etiology)
7. Herpes simplex virus (HSV) keratoconjunctivitis
8. Herpes zoster ophthalmicus

M. Streitz, MD
Department of Emergency Medicine, San Antonio Uniformed Services Health Education Consortium, San Antonio, TX, USA

© Springer International Publishing AG, part of Springer Nature 2018
B. Long, A. Koyfman (eds.), *Handbook of Emergency Ophthalmology*, https://doi.org/10.1007/978-3-319-78945-3_10

9. Corneal ulcer
10. Bacterial keratitis
11. Fungal keratitis
12. Uveitis/iritis
13. Endophthalmitis

Clinical Presentation

Patients present to the ED for eye-related concerns in a variety of ways. The emergency physician must evaluate for threats to life, limb, or eyesight. Common patient eye complaints include double or blurry vision, redness, pain, fever, discharge from the eye, foreign body sensation or foreign body in the eye, vision loss, color vision changes, floaters, and a "dark curtain," as well as redness, tenderness, or swelling of the structures around the eye. This chapter will discuss several common eye infections and disorders.

1. Periorbital cellulitis: Preseptal or periorbital cellulitis is an infection of the tissues anterior to the orbital septum and often presents with lid erythema, warmth to the touch, tenderness, and swelling, as well as low-grade fever (Fig. 10.1). The orbital septum is a thin fibrous membrane that divides the orbital from the preseptal compartments of the eye [1–6]. The Chandler classification system is used to categorize periorbital infections into five groups. This includes preseptal cellulitis as group 1, orbital cellulitis as group 2, and groups 3–5 which encompass subperiosteal orbital abscess, diffuse orbital infection or abscess, and cavernous sinus thrombosis, respectively [4–6]. Common routes for inoculation of pathogens causing periorbital cellulitis include direct inoculation following recent eyelid trauma and insect bites. Inoculation secondary to spread from contiguous structures such as the paranasal (particularly the ethmoid) sinuses, chalazia/hordeolum, impetigo, herpes simplex virus (HSV), and herpes zoster skin infection. Finally, hematogenous spread often secondary to an upper respiratory or middle ear infection can also cause preseptal

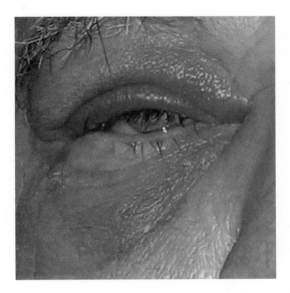

FIGURE 10.1 Preseptal cellulitis. Obtained from EyeRounds.Org on 20 Aug 2017

cellulitis [1–6]. Bacteria such as gram-positive cocci, i.e., *Staphylococcus* and *Streptococcus* species, are responsible for the vast majority of infections, and the strain depends on the route of infection. *Staphylococcus aureus* and *S. epidermidis* are common after penetrating injury, whereas *Streptococcus pneumoniae* is most common secondary to sinusitis [4–7]. Although much less common than before the introduction of the *Haemophilus influenzae* type b vaccine, those children under 5 years old who are unimmunized are still at increased risk for infection secondary to those bacteria [7]. Common viruses include adenovirus, HSV, and varicella zoster.

2. Orbital cellulitis: Orbital cellulitis occurs posterior to the orbital septum and involves the soft tissues found within the bony orbit [1, 2, 6] (Fig. 10.2). Again, similar to preseptal cellulitis, this is commonly due to spread from a local infection occurring in adjacent structures (>90% from

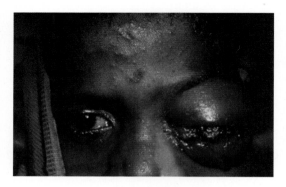

FIGURE 10.2 Orbital cellulitis. Obtained from EyeRounds.Org on 20 Aug 2017

underlying sinus disease). Odontogenic origins of infection are also possible if there is orbital involvement [6]. Both preseptal and orbital cellulitis have periorbital edema and erythema; however, unlike preseptal cellulitis, orbital cellulitis will commonly have proptosis, extraocular movement (EOM) restriction secondary to pain and swelling, diplopia, ophthalmoplegia, pain with eye movement, and patient toxicity on exam [1, 4–6, 8]. There is a greater risk of morbidity and mortality associated with orbital cellulitis as compared to preseptal cellulitis [6]. Bacterial infections in children are often due to a single organism, likely *S. aureus* or *S. pneumoniae* [1, 2, 5, 6]. Infections commonly are polymicrobial in adults and adolescents. The number of bacteria involved ranges from 2 to 5, and common organisms include *Streptococcus* and *Staphylococcus*. In the event of odontogenic etiology, *Peptostreptococcus* is commonly seen. Fungal and *Pseudomonas* infections may occur in immunocompromised patients [4, 6, 8].

3. Conjunctivitis: The spectrum of conjunctivitis encompasses infectious and noninfectious etiologies. Within infectious causes, bacterial, viral, and neonatal all deserve specific discussions. Other infectious causes include parasitic and

fungal but are much more rare. Included in noninfectious are allergic, chemical or toxic, and systemic, among many other causes that do not fall under the scope of this chapter. Conjunctivitis is an inflammation or infection of the conjunctiva and commonly presents with hyperemia, erythema, matting, a gritty or foreign body sensation, as well as edema and discharge from the eye [1, 2, 9–11]. The clinical presentations of bacterial, viral, and neonatal conjunctivitis have significant overlap and are often nonspecific [12, 13]. Visual acuity should be normal, and a recent history upper respiratory infection suggests viral cause. Of the 3% of ED visits related to ocular complaints, conjunctivitis accounts for over 30% [9]. Bacterial and viral are by far the most common etiologies of conjunctivitis with viral being the more common (80%) [14–18] of the two, despite bacterial being more common in children [1, 2, 14–19]. Risk factors for infection include contact with contaminated sources such as fingers, fomites, and oculogenital contact of an infected individual [9, 10, 19–22]. Anything that causes a disruption of the epithelial layer of the eye such as trauma and immunocompromised status also increases risk.

Bacterial conjunctivitis is characterized by an acute onset of symptoms with minimal to no pain and matting of the eyelids in the morning. The most common pathogens in children include nontypeable *H. influenzae*, *S. pneumoniae*, and *Moraxella catarrhalis* [23]. In adults, the most common microbes are *Staphylococcus* and *Streptococcus*, followed by *H. influenzae* [23]. The course lasts approximately 7–10 days [10]. Bacterial conjunctivitis is most prevalent in the months from December to April [19]. Incubation typically ranges from 1 to 7 days, and communicability ranges from 2 to 7 days [9, 10, 19]. Any patient presenting with signs and symptoms of 4 or more weeks has chronic bacterial conjunctivitis, and these patients are most commonly infected secondary to *Staphylococcus aureus*, *Moraxella lacunata*, and enteric bacteria.

Bacterial infections of note are those associated with sexually transmitted infections occurring due to oculogenital spread. *Neisseria gonorrhoeae* should be considered in hyperacute bacterial conjunctivitis, which presents with severe copious amounts of purulent ocular discharge and decreased vision. True *N. gonorrhoeae* involvement places the patient at risk for corneal perforation [10, 24]. Chlamydial conjunctivitis is not uncommon, with a prevalence ranging from 1.8 to 5.6% of cases [17]. Presentation is typically unilateral, and a concurrent genital infection is likely (54% of men and 74% of women) [11, 25]. Patients also present with a purulent or mucopurulent discharge, conjunctival hyperemia, and typically will have mild symptoms for months before presentation. Finally, conjunctivitis secondary to trachoma will be discussed. Trachoma is caused by the subtypes A through C of *Chlamydia trachomatis* and is the leading cause of blindness in the world [25, 26]. Mucopurulent discharge and pain are the most common presenting symptoms. Blindness is a late complication and is due to corneal, eyelid, and conjunctival scarring.

4. Viral conjunctivitis is comprised of two main entities: epidemic keratoconjunctivitis (EKC) and pharyngoconjunctival fever, both of which are typically secondary to adenoviruses (65–90%) and is considered highly contagious with a risk of transmission ranging from 10 to 50% [10, 19, 27, 28]. Incubation typically ranges from 5 to 12 days, and the communicability ranges from 10 to 14 days [9, 10, 19]. Viral conjunctivitis is most commonly seen in the summer. Pharyngoconjunctival fever is characterized by pharyngitis, high fever, preauricular lymphadenopathy (typically bilaterally), as well as bilateral conjunctivitis. EKC typically has unilateral lymphadenopathy and has a more severe presentation with increased discharge and hyperemia. Patients may also have symptoms of a recent upper respiratory infection.

5. Neonatal conjunctivitis, also known as neonatorum ophthalmia, is defined as conjunctival inflammation occurring

in the first 30 days of life and can be secondary to chemical, bacterial, and viral conjunctivitis. Treatment is important due to the potential for permanent scarring and blindness if left untreated. Although chemical conjunctivitis is not covered in depth here, it is important to note that the overall prevalence of chemical causes has decreased significantly since the abandonment of silver nitrate after delivery, making infectious causes much more likely in today's population. Common causes of bacterial conjunctivitis are *Chlamydia trachomatis* (most common), *Neisseria gonorrhoeae*, *S. aureus*, *Pseudomonas aeruginosa*, and *Streptococcus* species. Risk factors include maternal infections encountered during birth, inadequate prophylaxis at birth, premature rupture of membranes, ocular trauma during delivery, poor prenatal care, and poor hygienic conditions during delivery [1, 2, 29]. Chlamydial infections in the United States complicate 4–10% of pregnancies, and those infants of untreated mothers have a 30–40% chance of developing conjunctivitis. Timing of infections with regard to birth is important in the diagnosis of neonatal conjunctivitis. Infectious causes are not expected if less than 24 h of life. *N. gonorrhoeae* infections present 3–5 days after birth, and *C. trachomatis* presents in days 5–14 [1, 2, 29]. HSV can present in the first 1–2 weeks of life, and vesicles are likely present on examination.

6. Contact lens complications: Wearing contacts causes alterations to the eye through several mechanisms including trauma, decreased corneal oxygenation, decreased wetting/lubrication, allergic and inflammatory responses, and infection [30]. Symptom-related complications are no different than those already discussed with regard to the "red eye" and can present within 24 h after onset. Bacterial keratitis accounts for >90% of the infectious causes related to contact lens wearing. *Pseudomonas aeruginosa* is the most common pathogen, followed by *Staphylococcus*, *Streptococcus*, and *Serratia*. Although rare, fungal keratitis caused by *Acanthamoeba* is closely related to contact

lens use [30–33]. A major risk factor for bacterial keratitis in contact lens patients is corneal abrasions [34]. Even without abrasions, contact lenses place the patient at an increased risk, particularly with overnight or extended wear types [35–37]. Rates of infectious keratitis increase with the length of time each contact is used. Rigid lenses pose the least risk, while extended-wear soft lenses pose a 5× increase in risk [38]. Other risk factors include lens hygiene, poor supervision by an eye care professional, smoking, male gender, low socioeconomic status, and young age [39–42].

7. HSV keratoconjunctivitis: HSV involved conjunctivitis comprises 1.3–4.8% of acute conjunctivitis and is usually unilateral upon presentation [15–18]. It is a major cause of blindness secondary to corneal scarring worldwide, and HSV-1 accounts for most ocular infections, although HSV-2 is on the rise [43]. Ocular HSV-1 disease comprises eyelid lesions (herpetic blepharitis), conjunctivitis, keratitis (most common), retinitis, and rarely scleritis [44]. This most often seen in young adults and typically presents with a thin, watery discharge. Patients also have a foreign body sensation, possibly decreased visual acuity, tearing, and photophobia. On fluorescein exam, a dendritic pattern with terminal bulbs and/or punctate lesions can be seen. Risk factors for infection with ocular involvement include primary infections or recurrences of latent infection. Latent infections tend to involve the same eye [45, 46]. Other risk factors include immunosuppression and ultraviolet light exposure (laser treatment for corneal refractive surgery and environmental). The disease course runs over 1–2 weeks with appropriate treatment.

8. Herpes zoster ophthalmicus: Herpes zoster, the virus responsible for shingles, can also affect the eye. Reactivation of the varicella zoster virus along the trigeminal nerve (CN V) in the ophthalmic division leads to this condition and is present in 10–20% of reactivations [47]. Patients commonly present with painful palpation to the forehead and face, fever, hyperesthesia, redness, and

the typical unilateral vesicular rash. There may be vesicular lesions on the eyelid, particularly if the first and second branches of the nerve are involved. Hutchinson's sign is also seen and indicates that the nasociliary branch of the trigeminal nerve is involved. Eyelids and conjunctiva are involved in patients with shingles, 45.8% and 41.1%, respectively [10, 31]. Patients with zoster can have corneal complications (38.2%) and subsequent uveitis (19.1%) [10, 31]. The typical patient population includes adults >60 years old. Diagnosis and treatment are important to prevent acute necrotizing retinitis associated with the condition [1].

9. Corneal ulcer: Corneal ulcers are considered a type of keratitis and can be large or small, typically round, and are best visualized under slit-lamp examination where edema and a white clouding can be seen. Common causes are overuse of contact lenses. Patients typically present with pain, redness, vision changes depending on the location of the ulcer, and photophobia [1]. Infections associated with corneal ulcers can be bacterial, viral, fungal, or due to *Acanthamoeba* and are discussed further in the keratitis section of this chapter. They can have an acute and rapid presentation or a delayed presentation after a traumatic event. Thorough history usually helps delineate the cause.

10. Bacterial keratitis: Bacterial keratitis is a medical emergency and is often referred to as a "corneal ulcer" due to their strong association. Patients usually have at least one risk factor for the disease, with the predominant risk factor being contact lens wear. As discussed in contact lens complications, overnight wear, poor hygiene, infrequent lens changing, male sex, and low socioeconomic status also increase risk [39–42]. Bacterial keratitis can form in those without risk factors and is typically associated with virulent organisms such as *Neisseria*, *Diphtheria*, and *Listeria* species [48]. Patients will present with symptoms of redness, pain, photophobia, and an objective foreign body sensation, a sign of an active corneal process. Slit-lamp and fluorescein findings include a corneal infiltrate/

opacity with a focal hazy or cloudy appearance to them. Frequently, a corneal ulcer with fluorescein uptake is seen. In severe cases, a hypopyon, a layer of white blood cells in the anterior chamber, may be visible [49–51].

11. Fungal keratitis: Fungal keratitis is a common disease worldwide but is rare in the United States. The incidence varies widely based on the geographic region of the United States. It represents 2% of the keratitis cases in New York and upwards of 35% in Florida [50]. Risk factors for fungal keratitis include trauma, particularly trauma with vegetative material (tree branches, soils, and grasses), soft contact lens use, topical corticosteroid use, and immunosuppression [50]. Patients present with symptoms similar to bacterial and viral keratitis (pain, photophobia, foreign body sensation, and blurred vision) but with a more insidious onset. Patients returning to the ED for a corneal ulcer that has not responded to broad-spectrum antibiotics should raise suspicion. Examination with a slit lamp and fluorescein reveals a corneal infiltrate or ulcer. Fungal corneal infections in the Southern United States (i.e., Florida), the *Fusarium* spp., are the most common cause (45–76%), whereas in the northern states (i.e., New York, North Dakota), *Candida* and *Aspergillus* spp. are more common [50, 52]. Without prompt diagnosis and treatment, there are devastating consequences for patients.

12. Uveitis/iritis: Anterior uveitis describes inflammation of the iris and/or the ciliary body. Inflammation of the iris alone is iritis, while inflammation of the iris and ciliary body is iridocyclitis. Anterior uveitis accounts for over 90% of the patients diagnosed with uveitis and 10–15% of cases of blindness in the United States [53]. Iritis can be caused by a wide variety of inciting events/conditions. Trauma, systemic and ocular infections, autoimmune diseases (adult and juvenile rheumatoid arthritis, sarcoidosis, and ankylosing spondylitis), and immunosuppression are other causes [1]. Ocular infections include keratitis, cytomegalovirus (CMV) retinitis secondary to AIDS [1], and

systemic infections secondary to Epstein-Barr virus, influenza, and syphilis [54, 55]. Patients typically present with severe eye pain but rarely have discharge.

13. Endophthalmitis: Endophthalmitis is a severe infection of the anterior, posterior, and vitreous chambers found within the globe (Fig. 10.3). It is most commonly found after penetrating trauma to the eye but also occurs secondary to hematogenous spread of immunocompromised patients and after routine eye surgery or procedures (cataracts and injections) [1, 56, 57]. Patients present with acute onset painful and red eye with decreased visual acuity and approximately 85% have a hypopyon. Postsurgical and postinjection endophthalmitis commonly present within a week of the procedure, typically symptom-free until about 24 h prior to presentation. Endogenous spread is associated with endocarditis in 40% of patients and can also occur secondary to abscesses, UTI, and meningitis [56]. Common bacteria include *Staphylococcus*, *Streptococcus*, and *Bacillus* [1, 56]. Fungal and mold endophthalmitis, although rare, are typically from an endogenous and exogenous source, respectively. Risk factors for fungal infections include immunosuppression, indwelling central venous catheters, total parenteral nutrition, neutropenia,

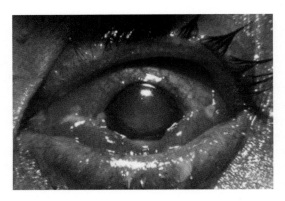

FIGURE 10.3 Endophthalmitis. Obtained from EyeRounds.Org on 20 Aug 2017

recent gastrointestinal surgery or perforation, and recent broad-spectrum antibiotics. *Candida* is the main cause [56, 58]. Mold infections (*Aspergillus*) are most typically secondary to penetrating trauma, after eye surgery, or progressing fungal keratitis [56].

Differential Diagnosis

There is a broad differential diagnosis for eye infections, as redness, swelling, and tenderness of the eyelid encompasses a vast differential. The differential for those "red eye" complaints includes cellulitis (septal and preseptal), dacryocystitis, chalazion, hordeolum (stye), dacryoadenitis, anaphylaxis, conjunctivitis, keratitis, and endophthalmitis. Other, more specific eyelid diagnoses include cysts, carcinoma, xanthelasma, papilloma, pyogenic granuloma, retinoblastoma, amyloid deposition, and any skin condition that can be found elsewhere on the body can be found on the eyelid [8, 12, 59]. This chapter will discuss eye infections, but noninfectious etiology must also be considered such as thyroid eye disease, blunt trauma, and autoimmune inflammatory diseases.

Evaluation

A solid understanding of eye anatomy provides a solid foundation for the evaluation of any eye complaint. A thorough evaluation of optic nerve function and ocular motility can provide a vast amount of useful clinical information. The exam should include best-corrected visual acuity, color vision assessment, visual field testing, fluorescein staining with a Wood's lamp exam, papillary function (particularly evaluating for afferent papillary defect), and EOM testing, as well as intraocular pressure (IOP) in the ED [6, 8, 9]. A comprehensive review of systems should be obtained. A history of photophobia, foreign body sensation, and visual changes should be elicited. Screening for trauma, contact lens wear, and any inflammatory or autoimmune disorders is needed. The specific evaluation and physical exam findings for the specific conditions are as follows:

1. Preseptal cellulitis: Hallmarks of physical exam include periorbital edema and erythema (Fig. 10.1). Warmth to the touch, tenderness, and swelling as well as low-grade fever are also common presenting symptoms. The absence of proptosis, pain with EOM, vision loss, and diplopia is required. Pupillary function as well as color vision should be intact [6]. If any of these are abnormal, then orbital involvement is highly likely. If patients have high fever or if fever is increasing, blood cultures should be obtained [5].

2. Orbital cellulitis: Fever, leukocytosis, afferent papillary defect, proptosis, EOM dysfunction, and vision loss should increase suspicion for orbital involvement and prompt rapid treatment (Fig. 10.2). An afferent papillary defect indicates optic nerve involvement. If orbital cellulitis is high on the differential, then a thin-slice non-contrasted orbital CT scan is the modality of choice, providing information not only on the orbit but surrounding tissue and structures of interest [1, 2, 5, 6, 8].

3. Bacterial conjunctivitis: Both viral and bacterial conjunctivitis can present with either bilateral or unilateral eye involvement. Bacterial conjunctivitis presents with red eye and mucopurulent or purulent discharge, as well as chemosis. Bilateral matting with adherence of the eyelids in the morning and lack of itching is a high predictor for bacterial over viral pathology [19]. See Chap. 6 for picture.

4. Viral conjunctivitis: Patients often report a recent URI when asked. Itching, a slower progression or appearance of symptoms, and a mucoid or watery discharge are more common with viral presentations. Preauricular lymphadenopathy may be present. See Chap. 6 for picture.

5. Neonatal conjunctivitis: Timing is critical in the neonate presenting with concerns for conjunctivitis. Prenatal care, care at delivery (silver nitrate vs. erythromycin), and maternal history (STI's) are also important when examining the

patient. Chlamydial infection can present with mild conjunctival injection and tearing coupled with a mucopurulent discharge and a pseudomembrane [30]. Neisseria infections present more acutely, with sever lid edema and a copious mucopurulent discharge and are the most feared infection in the eye. Any ill-appearing neonate should raise suspicion for systemic illness and should prompt a full sepsis workup. Chemical irritant conjunctivitis is typically seen in the first 48 h of life commonly secondary to silver nitrate as topical prophylaxis. See Chap. 6 for further discussion, as well as for picture.

6. Contact lens complications: Bacterial keratitis, the most common infection related to contact lens use, typically presents with symptoms in 24 h. Most commonly patients present with redness, decreased vision concerns, and photophobia and on exam will have corneal uptake with fluorescein. Patients with keratitis can present with a hypopyon or white blood cells in the anterior chamber. Hypopyon is found more frequently in cases secondary to fungal infection. Other exam findings can be stromal loss, stromal infiltrates, and corneal edema. Stromal infiltrates tend to be yellow in bacterial keratitis and white if fungal in nature [51, 52]. See Chap. 6 for picture.

7. HSV keratoconjunctivitis: This disease presents with edematous and ecchymotic eyelids, and frequently there are eyelid or bulbar conjunctival vesicles or ulcers. On slit-lamp exam, there can be punctate and dendritic lesions [1, 2, 39]. Discharge is typically serosanguinous or nonpurulent. For neonates, vesicles on the skin surrounding the eye and involvement of the corneal epithelium are important to distinguish from other forms of keratitis or conjunctivitis [39]. See Chap. 6 for picture.

8. Herpes zoster ophthalmicus: There may be vesicular lesions on the eyelid if the first and second branches of the trigeminal nerve are involved. Hutchinson's sign (vesicles on the tip of the nose) highly correlates to ocular involvement (76% of patients). Pseudodendritic lesions can be seen on exam with fluorescein [1]. See Chap. 6 for picture.

9. Corneal ulcer: Corneal infiltrates can be seen on either direct visualization or with the aid of a slit lamp and appear as a white opacity on the cornea. Ulcers tend to be round on examination with or without fluorescein. See Chap. 6 for picture.

10. Bacterial keratitis: Patients with bacterial keratitis may or may not have affected vision, but this condition typically produces objective findings of foreign body sensation (inability to keep eye open) and photophobia. The pupil may be miotic at 1–2 mm [34, 38, 39, 49]. On exam, a corneal opacity is frequently seen as well as conjunctival injection. Fulminant cases of keratitis may present with a hypopyon. See Chap. 6 for picture.

11. Fungal keratitis: Providers must have a high index of suspicion for nonbacterial keratitis. A thorough clinical history, clinical exam, and attempting to isolate the specific organism are of the utmost importance. Tropical climates coupled with trauma, no matter how benign appearing, place a patient at increased risk for a fungal infection [52]. Fungal keratitis may demonstrate a feathery edge to the ulcer, whereas a lesion secondary to yeast is more defined. Satellite lesions may also be present and should increase concerns for a fungal infection, as should the presence of a hypopyon. Diagnosis will not be made in the ED, as this requires specialized corneal scrapings/punch biopsy and cultures for confirmation [52, 58]. A corneal defect is typically seen 24–36 h after injury [58]. See Chap. 6 for picture.

12. Uveitis/iritis: On exam, there can be significant conjunctival injection, most prominent at the limbus (aka ciliary flush). There is a lack of discharge, and patients do not usually have a foreign body sensation [49]. The pupil, on exam, can be miotic (1–2 mm) and sluggish when reacting to light. Consensual photophobia is common [15, 52]. On slit-lamp exam, providers may see cell and flare, which is white blood cells and protein in the anterior chamber. See Chap. 6 for picture.

13. Endophthalmitis: Examination reveals decreased visual acuity, hazy or opaque appearance to the infected chamber,

hyperemia of the conjunctiva, and chemosis. One review finds 94.3% of patients reported blurred vision, 8.1% complained of a red eye, and 74% reported pain upon presentation [57]. Visual acuity is important when discussing the case with the ophthalmologist, and differentiating hand motion (HM) and light perception (LP) are considered the most important in the evaluation [57].

Management

1. Preseptal cellulitis: Understanding the mechanism of injury and initiating antibiotics covering the most likely pathogen are essential in the management of preseptal cellulitis. Broad-spectrum antibiotics covering gram-positive and gram-negative bacteria must be prescribed. *Staphylococcus* and *Streptococcus* species are the primary causes of preseptal cellulitis for puncture wounds, and anaerobes predominate in the cause secondary to human bites. Oral antibiotics can be used for the majority of patients with close follow-up to ensure clinical improvement. Oral antibiotic options include amoxicillin/clavulanate 875/125 mg every 12 h (children at a dose of amoxicillin 90 mg/kg/day and for clavulanate 6.4 mg/kg/day divided in two doses), levofloxacin 500–700 mg IV or PO every 24 h, and azithromycin >6 m/o is 10 mg/kg and in adults 250–500 mg every 24 h PO [6]. For infections secondary to eyelid trauma, coverage for gram-positive (*Staphylococcus*) includes dicloxacillin (pediatric dosing is 12.5–25 mg/kg every 6 h for <40 kg weight, and for over 40 kg, the dosing is the same as adults at 125–250 mg every 6 h), flucloxacillin, and first-generation cephalosporins such as cephalexin (25–50 mg/kg/day divided every 6 h and for adults 250–1000 mg every 6 h) and cefazolin (pediatric dosing is 50 mg/kg every 8 h and for adults, 1 g every 8 h). Intravenous antibiotic choices include third-generation cephalosporins such as ceftriaxone (50–100 mg/kg/day divided in 12–24 h dosing and for adults

1–2 g every 24 h), cefotaxime (pediatrics 150–200 mg/kg/ day every 6–8 h with a max dose of 12 g/day and for adults 1–2 g every 4–6 h), and ceftazidime (1 m/o to 12 y/o 90–150 mg/kg/day divided every 8 h and for adults 1 g every 8–12 h) [6]. Ampicillin/sulbactam (pediatrics 50 mg/ kg, and for adults 1.5–3 g as well every 6 h IV) is also an option. Community-associated methicillin-resistant *S. aureus* (MRSA) can typically be adequately treated with oral regimens of trimethoprim-sulfamethoxazole (for pediatrics sulfamethoxazole at 40 mg/kg/day divided every 12 h and for trimethoprim 8 mg/kg/day divided every 12 h; adults are dosed 160 mg oral or 2.5 mg/kg IV every 12 h) or clindamycin (pediatric dosing 8–16 mg/kg/ day divided every 6–8 h and for adults 300–450,450 mg PO every 6 h or 600–900 mg IV every 8 h) [6]. Hospital-associated MRSA should be covered with intravenous vancomycin (for 1 m/o to 12 y/o 10 to 15 mg/kg/day and for patients >70 kg, 1 g IV) or oral linezolid (<12 y/o at 10 mg/kg and for adults 600 mg every 12 h). Trauma resulting in a penetrating injury with organic material or a human bite should have treatment that includes coverage for anaerobic organisms. Metronidazole (500 mg IV every 8 h) and clindamycin (same dose as above) or levofloxacin (750 mg IV every 24 h) should be adequate [1, 2, 6]. If an abscess is present, incision and drainage by ophthalmology for adequate treatment is recommended. Ensure tetanus is up to date. If patients present to the ED on outpatient oral antibiotic therapy and there is no improvement in the past 48 h or if there is evidence of extension of the infection, intravenous antibiotics should be started and CT scan obtained [6].

2. Orbital cellulitis: Prompt treatment is vital to successful treatment of orbital cellulitis. Broad-spectrum antibiotic coverage for the most likely organisms is the standard. For patients with suspected MRSA, the coverage includes vancomycin (15–20 mg/kg every 6 h for adults and 10–15 mg/kg every 6 h with a max dose of 4 g/day in children) or clindamycin (8–16 mg/kg/day divided every 6–8 h

in children and for adults, 300–450 mg PO every 6 h or 600–900 mg IV every 8 h) [6]. Once cultures are resulted and if the organism is MSSA, vancomycin should be stopped, and the regimen should be changed to nafcillin or oxacillin (both can be dosed at 2 g IV every 4 h for adults, and for children, dosing is 50–200 mg/kg/day every 4–6 h with a max dose of 12 g/day) [5]. Other antibiotic choices include ampicillin-sulbactam, ticarcillin-clavulanate (3 g IV every 4 h in adults and 200–300 mg/kg of ticarcillin every 4–6 h for pediatrics with a max dose if 18 g), piperacillin-tazobactam (4.5 g every 6 h for adults and 240 mg/kg/day every 8 h for pediatrics), ceftriaxone, and cefotaxime [5, 6]. Combination therapy with a broad-spectrum cephalosporin along with metronidazole or clindamycin for anaerobic coverage is typical. If fungal cellulitis is a clinical concern, amphotericin B (1 mg/kg IV q24h) or voriconazole (6 mg/kg IV q12h for two doses, then 4 mg/kg IV q12h) are first-line choices. Patients with orbital cellulitis secondary to sinusitis may be candidates for surgical drainage, but this would be best managed in consultation with subspecialists as needed.

3. Bacterial conjunctivitis: While most cases are self-limiting, cases secondary to highly virulent bacteria such as *S. pneumoniae*, *N. gonorrhoeae*, and *H. influenzae* benefit from treatment [60]. There are no major advantages to the available broad-spectrum antibiotics available, but resistance patterns differ in specific regions of the United States. A newer antibiotic besifloxacin (1 gtt every 8 h) shows promise for increased rates of clinical resolution and can be used with suspected bacterial conjunctivitis [61]. Common antibiotic drops include polymyxin combination drugs, aminoglycosides, or fluoroquinolones (ciprofloxacin (1–2 gtt every 6 h or ointment every 8 h, ofloxacin (1–2 gtt every 6 h), levofloxacin (1–2 gtt every 6 h), moxifloxacin (every 8 h), or gatifloxacin (every 8 h)) [19]. Other drugs include bacitracin or ciprofloxacin ointment. Dosing for each of the antibiotics in four times a day over 5–7 days. Topical steroids should be avoided.

If *N. gonorrhoeae* is of concern, 1 g of ceftriaxone should be provided. Patients should be treated for concurrent chlamydial infection with either azithromycin 1 g orally or doxycycline 100 mg twice daily for 7 days [60]. *Chlamydia trachomatis* subtypes A and C should be treated with a single dose of oral azithromycin 20 mg/kg. Antibiotic regimens of tetracycline or erythromycin for 6 weeks topically or orally for 3 weeks can be used [19].

4. Viral conjunctivitis: Treatment is mainly supportive. Patients should receive teaching about cold compresses and be provided decongestants, artificial tears, and strict return precautions. Antihistamines can also be of use for symptom relief. A key point is prevention of coinfection of the other eye.

5. Neonatal conjunctivitis: Patients with concerns for *N. gonorrhoeae* infections require eye irrigation, intravenous penicillin G 100 Ku/kg/day in four divided doses, penicillin G benzathine 50 ku/kg/day, or ceftriaxone 50 mg/kg IM as a single dose for 7 days. They should also receive bacitracin or erythromycin ointment every 2–4 h [39]. For chlamydial infections, erythromycin eye drops four times a day plus erythromycin liquid 50 mg/kg/day in four divided doses for 2–3 weeks is recommended.

6. Contact lens complications: Conjunctivitis and keratitis (fungal and bacterial) are the most common infectious complications of wear. See those sections for specific treatment. Of note, a pathogen that is closely related to contact lens use is *Acanthamoeba*, and upwards of 90% of patients with this infection wear contacts. Specific treatment for *Acanthamoeba* keratitis is polyhexamethylene biguanide, propamidine isethionate, and neomycin [39, 62].

7. HSV keratoconjunctivitis: This is usually a self-limiting process, but patients should be referred and evaluated within several days by an ophthalmologist for confirmation of diagnosis and monitoring [49]. A review of over 100 trials found four antiviral agents including trifluridine, acyclovir, ganciclovir, and brivudine to be equally

effective, resulting in over 90% cure rate in 2 weeks [63]. Treatment options include acyclovir intravenous at 45 mg/kg/day plus vidarabine 3% ointment five times a day for 14–21 days depending on the presence or absence of any central nervous system involvement [19]. Acyclovir can also be administered as a topical or oral agent. There is a 3% ointment in 200, 400, or 800 mg formulations. Treatment includes five times a day dosing for 10 days. Oral suspension includes a 200 mg/5 mL suspension and is dosed 400 mg five times a day for 10 days [19, 51, 60, 64]. There is also a dermatologic ointment, 5% applied six times a day for 7 days. Ganciclovir is available at a 0.15% ophthalmic gel applied five times a day until the epithelium heals and then three times a day for 7 days [19, 65]. Trifluridine 1% is given one drop every 2 h or eight to nine times a day for the first week and is typically tapered [51, 66]. Valacyclovir, oral at 500 mg three times a day for 7–10 days, is an option [60]. Topical corticosteroids are not recommended due to the potential for harm [19].

8. Zoster ophthalmicus: Patients can be treated with oral antivirals including acyclovir 800 mg five times a day for 7–10 days or famciclovir 500 mg three times a day for 7–10 days. Valacyclovir 1 g oral three times a day can also be used [19, 51].

9. Corneal ulcer: Specific treatments for suppurative corneal ulcer infections are discussed in the keratitis sections, both fungal and bacterial. In one institution, 71.9% of cultures of corneal ulcers were culture positive for bacterial, fungal, and parasitic [62]. These infections need to be treated.

10. Bacterial keratitis: If patients have not already done so, they need to remove contact lenses as soon as possible, as overnight wear of lenses is the single greatest risk factor [1, 34, 38, 39]. Patients should have topical antibiotics started immediately, though preferentially after cultures are obtained [49]. All patients should have an emergent ophthalmologic consultation for scrapings and culture of infection [2]. If ophthalmology is not readily available,

broad-spectrum topical antibiotics should be started. Options include a fluoroquinolone (ofloxacin, moxifloxacin, gatifloxacin, or ciprofloxacin) or combination therapy with cephalosporin and aminoglycoside [2, 48]. Approximately 95% of infections will respond to appropriately chosen initial antibiotics; therefore, culture results are often unnecessary [48]. Cycloplegics can offer symptom relief, as this decreases pain secondary to ciliary spasms. If an ulcer with epithelial defects is found, ophthalmic fluoroquinolones every hour around the clock are recommended [51]. Ulcers that are large and vision-threatening should be treated with fortified tobramycin or gentamicin (15 mg/mL) every hour around the clock alternating with fortified vancomycin (25 mg/mL).

11. Fungal keratitis: Treatment options are limited, and medical treatment fails in approximately 15–20% of cases [67, 68]. Surgical intervention is required in 15–40% of cases [68, 69]. The emergency physician will not definitively diagnose or treat this disease, but it is important to consider the disease when risk factors or physical findings consistent with the disease are present. Emergent referral to an ophthalmologist may lead to earlier diagnosis and treatment and decrease rates of medical failure [50]. Natamycin 5% is the only FDA-approved topical ocular antibiotic. Amphotericin B is also an option in a 0.15% dilution. Miconazole (topical suspension 1%, topical cream 2%, subconjunctival 5–10 mg), ketoconazole (topical 5%, oral 300 mg/day), clotrimazole (topical 1%), fluconazole (topical 0.2%, oral 200 mg/day), itraconazole (topical 1%, oral 100–200 mg twice daily), and voriconazole (topical 1%, oral, 200 mg twice a day) are recommended drugs with variable activity. Voriconazole has the broadest coverage of the azole medication family [52].

12. Uveitis/iritis: The mainstay of treatment is long-acting cycloplegic medications such as homatropine to aid in pain control by blocking papillary constriction [54].

13. Endophthalmitis: This is a true ophthalmologic emergency, and patients require ophthalmologist evaluation

as soon as possible. Intravitreal antibiotics are the definitive treatment and commonly require a second dose 24–48 h after the first treatment. Intravitreal vancomycin 1 g and ceftazidime 2.25 mg are the empirical antibiotics most commonly use in the United States. Amikacin 0.4 mg is used in the event of a cephalosporin allergy. Gatifloxacin and moxifloxacin are also used in a concentration of 400 mcg/0.1 mL, and if concerned for fungal etiology, amphotericin B, 5–10 mcg/0.1 mL, is recommended [56, 58]. Itraconazole, voriconazole, and fluconazole are treatment options for fungal causes, with treatment lasting for months. Patients may require operative treatment for a vitrectomy, which is a debridement of the vitreous, leading to improved visual outcomes [56, 57]. Systemic antibiotics are of little help, as they penetrate the aqueous too slowly to reach adequate concentrations. The only exception to that is moxifloxacin which reaches adequate intraocular levels [56]. Corticosteroids are controversial, and their use should be in conjunction with ophthalmology.

Disposition

1. Periorbital cellulitis: Disposition depends on several factors including age, clinical appearance, reliability of patients and parents for children, and ability to obtain follow-up. Children under 1 year of age and those more severe cases should receive intravenous antibiotics and hospital observation [5]. The recommended duration of therapy is 7–10 days, and if there are any signs of local cellulitis, oral antibiotics should be continued until all erythema has resolved [5].
2. Orbital cellulitis: Delayed treatment and management of the infection can lead to a significant morbidity for the patient, including blindness, orbital apex syndrome (comprised of ophthalmoplegia, blepharoptosis, decreased corneal sensation, and vision loss), cavernous sinus

thrombosis, cranial nerve palsies, meningitis, intracranial abscesses, and even death [5, 6]. All children and the majority of adults with orbital cellulitis should be admitted to the hospital. Intravenous antibiotic treatment should continue for a minimum of 3 days (clinical improvement should be evident), and then oral antibiotic therapy should continue for a total treatment course of 10–21 days [5]. Candidates for surgical intervention include those who are not responding to treatment or are worsening despite treatment, decreased visual acuity, patients who develop an APD, and finally those who have an abscess. Conveying this information to the Ophthalmologist will help with disposition.

3. Bacterial conjunctivitis: Patients can be discharged home with medical and supportive therapies and recommendations to follow up with their primary doctor in 2–3 days to confirm resolution of symptoms. Artificial tears can aid with overall discomfort. Cold, moist compresses can decrease swelling. Decongestants have vasoconstrictive effects and can control pruritus for some patients. Saline irrigation of the affected eye can help with discomfort as well. Major teaching points for all forms of conjunctivitis include handwashing frequently, avoiding contact with either eye to prevent cross contamination, and avoiding sharing of cosmetics or towels [18, 60]. Neisserial infections should be viewed as an ocular finding of a systemic disease, and ophthalmologic consultation is essential [18]. Admission to a hospital for intravenous antibiotics should be considered based on clinical appearance.

4. Viral conjunctivitis: Patients can be discharged home with medical and supportive therapies and recommendations to follow up with their primary doctor in 7–10 days to confirm resolution of symptoms. Artificial tears can aid with overall discomfort. Cold, moist compresses can decrease swelling. Decongestants have vasoconstrictive effects and can control pruritus for some patients. Major teaching points for all forms of conjunctivitis include

handwashing frequently, avoiding contact with either eye to prevent cross contamination, and avoiding sharing of cosmetics or towels.

5. Neonatal conjunctivitis: Infants with evidence of or concern for chlamydial conjunctivitis require systemic antibiotics due to a prevalence of over 50% of patient can have concurrent genital tract, lung, and nasopharyngeal involvement. Hospitalization is recommended for both chlamydial and gonococcal infections [1, 2, 39].

6. Contact lens complications: Close evaluation and follow-up with ophthalmology is warranted as the clinical course should be followed for at least 48 h to ensure improvement once treatment is started [39].

7. Herpes simplex virus (HSV) keratoconjunctivitis: Patients should be started on topical and oral antivirals to help shorten the course of the disease [1, 2, 39, 60]. Close follow-up with ophthalmology is warranted.

8. Zoster ophthalmicus: Hutchinson's sign (vesicles on the tip of the nose) highly correlates to involvement of the cornea and warrants a referral to ophthalmology with close follow-up and reevaluation.

9. Corneal ulcer: Most ulcers need to be seen by ophthalmology within 24 h. If infection is involved, they can rapidly lead to opacification and vision loss [1].

10. Bacterial keratitis: Concern for this diagnosis warrants a same day evaluation by an ophthalmologist, particularly if a hypopyon is present, as this finding is often associated with infectious keratitis or endophthalmitis [49]. The eye should not be patched, as this facilitates spread of infection. Further follow-up and surgical vs. medical management will be further determined by the specialist. Daily follow-up with evaluation should be instituted until a response is noted to the treatment regimen.

11. Fungal keratitis: Clinical suspicion for this diagnosis or a hypopyon on exam warrants a same day evaluation by an ophthalmologist, as it is often associated with infectious keratitis or endophthalmitis [49]. Further follow-up and surgical vs. medical management will be further determined by the specialist.

12. Uveitis/iritis: Isolated iritis without an apparent cause and no clear autoimmune condition should be evaluated by an ophthalmologist in 24–48 h [2].
13. Endophthalmitis: A hypopyon on exam warrants a same day evaluation by an ophthalmologist, as it is often associated with infectious keratitis or endophthalmitis [49]. Ophthalmology will drive the ultimate disposition, but patients will need close follow-up as reinjection of intravitreal antibiotics is frequently needed, as is surgery [56, 57]. Patient outcomes such as visual acuity long-term are difficult to predict.

Pearls/Pitfalls

An incomplete physical examination, particularly a visual acuity with the addition of a slit-lamp examination, is a major pitfall with treatment of the above conditions. Other pitfalls are not adequately covering for the likely bacteria responsible for each condition and inadequate or untimely ophthalmology referral and evaluation.

Patients with foul smelling discharge with preseptal cellulitis are more likely to have an anaerobic infection [70].

In diabetics, alcoholics, and immunocompromised patients, mucormycosis must be considered, which requires extensive debridement. A black eschar may also be seen on the roof of the mouth or in the nose [70].

An infected eye should never be patched.

Dendrites on slit-lamp examination can be seen in cytomegalovirus and adenovirus, not just with herpes simplex or herpes zoster infections [70].

Many of the bacteria that can cause conjunctivitis in an infant can lead to sepsis and death in that age group, and a full workup should be considered.

Failure to recognize a patient with both genital and ocular symptoms as a potential gonococcal infection can have disastrous implications for a patient, as within 48 h untreated *N. gonorrhoeae* can penetrate the cornea.

Postoperative endophthalmitis can occur weeks to years after surgery.

References

1. Marx JA, Rosen P. Rosen's emergency medicine: concepts and clinical practice. 8th ed. Philadelphia, PA: Elsevier/Saunders; 2014. Chapter 71.
2. Walker RA, Adhikari S. Eye emergencies. In: Tintinalli's emergency medicine: a comprehensive study guide. 8th ed. New York: McGraw-Hill Education; 2016. p. 1543–78.
3. Chanmugan A, Bissonette A, Desai S, Putman S. Infectious disease emergencies. Chapter 15 – Periorbital infections. Oxford: Oxford University Press; 2016.
4. Mukherjee B, Yuen H. Emergencies of the orbit and adnexa. Berlin: Springer; 2016.
5. Hakim A. Eyelid and orbital infections. https://www.intechopen. com/books/advances-in-ophthalmology/orbital-cellulitis.
6. Pelton RW, Klapper SR. Focal points clinical modules for ophthalmologists: preseptal and orbital cellulitis. American Academy of Ophthalmology. 2008; 26(11).
7. Ambati BK, Ambati J, Azar N, et al. Periorbital and orbital cellulitis before and after the advent of Haemophilus influenzae type B vaccination. Ophthalmology. 2000;107:1450–3.
8. Mawn LA.Orbital cellulitis. http://eyewiki.org/Orbital_Cellulitis. Accessed 12 Apr 2017.
9. Azari AA, Barney NP. Conjunctivitis. JAMA. 2013;310(16):1721–9. https://doi.org/10.1001/jama.2013.280318.
10. Silverman MA, Brenner BE. "Acute conjunctivitis": overview, clinical evaluation, bacterial conjunctivitis. Web. 26 April 2016.
11. Leibowitz HM. The red eye. N Engl J Med. 2000;343(5):345–51.
12. Rietveld RP, van Weert HC, ter Riet G, Bindels PJ. Diagnostic impact of signs and symptoms in acute infectious conjunctivitis: systematic literature search. BMJ. 2003;327(7418):789.
13. Rietveld RP, ter Riet G, Bindels PJ, Sloos JH, van Weert HC. Predicting bacterial cause in infectious conjunctivitis. BMJ. 2004;329(7459):206–10.
14. Stenson S, Newman R, Fedukowicz H. Laboratory studies in acute conjunctivitis. Arch Ophthalmol. 1982;100(8):1275–7.
15. RoÅNnnerstam R, Persson K, Hansson H, Renmarker K. Prevalence of chlamydial eye infection in patients attending an eye clinic, a VD clinic, and in healthy persons. Br J Ophthalmol. 1985;69(5):385–8.

16. Harding SP, Mallinson H, Smith JL, Clearkin LG. Adult follicular conjunctivitis and neonatal ophthalmia in a Liverpool eye hospital, 1980-1984. Eye (Lond). 1987;1(pt 4):512–21.

17. Uchio E, Takeuchi S, Itoh N, et al. Clinical and epidemiological features of acute follicular conjunctivitis with special reference to that caused by herpes simplex virus type 1. Br J Ophthalmol. 2000;84(9):968–72.

18. Woodland RM, Darougar S, Thaker U, et al. Causes of conjunctivitis and keratoconjunctivitis in Karachi, Pakistan. Trans R Soc Trop Med Hyg. 1992;86(3):317–20.

19. Hovding G. Acute bacterial conjunctivitis. Acta Ophthalmol. 2008;86(1):5–17.

20. American Academy of Ophthalmology. Cornea/external disease panel. Preferred practice pattern guidelines: conjunctivitis-limited revision. San Francisco, CA: American Academy of Ophthalmology; 2011.

21. Sattar SA, Dimock KD, Ansari SA, Springthorpe VS. Spread of acute hemorrhagic conjunctivitis due to enterovirus-70: effect of air temperature and relative humidity on virus survival on fomites. J Med Virol. 1988;25(3):289–96.

22. Azar MJ, Dhaliwal DK, Bower KS, et al. Possible consequences of shaking hands with your patients with epidemic keratoconjunctivitis. Am J Ophthalmol. 1996;121(6):711–2.

23. Epling J, Smucny J. Bacterial conjunctivitis. Clin Evid. 2005;2(14):756–61.

24. Tarabishy AB, Jeng BH. Bacterial conjunctivitis: a review for internists. Cleve Clin J Med. 2008;75(7):507–12.

25. Postema EJ, Remeijer L, van der Meijden WI. Epidemiology of genital chlamydial infections in patients with chlamydial conjunctivitis. Genitourin Med. 1996;72(3):203–5.

26. Kumaresan JA, Mecaskey JW. The global elimination of blinding trachoma: progress and promise. Am J Trop Med Hyg. 2003;69(5_suppl):24–8.

27. Kaufman HE. Adenovirus advances: new diagnostic and therapeutic options. Curr Opin Ophthalmol. 2011;22(4):290–3.

28. O'Brien TP, Jeng BH, McDonald M, Raizman MB. Acute conjunctivitis: truth and misconceptions. Curr Med Res Opin. 2009;25(8):1953–61.

29. Bowman KM. Neonatal conjunctivitis. http://eyewiki.aao.org/Neonatal_Conjunctivitis. Accessed 27 Apr 2017.

30. Feldman BH, Rangel RA. Contact lens complications. http://eyewiki.org/Contact_lens_complications. Accessed 4 May 2017.

31. Huang AJ, Wichiensin P, Yang M. Bacterial keratitis. In: Krachmer JH, McMannis MJ, Holland EJ, editors. Cornea, vol. 1. 2nd ed. Philadelphia: Elsevier Mosby; 2005.

32. Mondino BJ, Weissman BA, Farb MD, Pettit TH. Corneal ulcers associated with daily-wear and extended-wear contact lenses. Am J Ophthalmol. 1986;102:58.

33. Puri LR, Shrestha GB, Shah DN, Chaudhary M, Thakur A. Ocular manifestations in herpes zoster ophthalmicus. Nepal J Ophthalmol. 2011;3(2):165–71.

34. Cope JR, Collier SA, Rao MM, et al. Contact lens wearer demographics and risk Behaviors for contact lens-related eye infections – United States, 2014. MMWR Morb Mortal Wkly Rep. 2015;64:865.

35. Chalmers RL, Wagner H, Mitchell GL, et al. Age and other risk factors for corneal infiltrative and inflammatory events in young soft contact lens wearers from the contact lens assessment in youth (CLAY) study. Invest Ophthalmol Vis Sci. 2011;52:6690.

36. Liesegang TJ. Contact lens-related microbial keratitis: part I: epidemiology. Cornea. 1997;16:125.

37. Thomas PA, Geraldine P. Infectious keratitis. Curr Opin Infect Dis. 2007;20:129.

38. Schein OD, Buehler PO, Stamler JF, et al. The impact of overnight wear on the risk of contact lens-associated ulcerative keratitis. Arch Ophthalmol. 1994;112:186.

39. Lee SY, Kim YH, Johnson D, et al. Contact lens complications in an urgent-care population: the University of California, Los Angeles, contact lens study. Eye Contact Lens. 2012;38:49.

40. Keay L, Stapleton F, Schein O. Epidemiology of contact lens-related inflammation and microbial keratitis: a 20-year perspective. Eye Contact Lens. 2007;33:346.

41. Keay L, Edwards K, Naduvilath T, et al. Microbial keratitis predisposing factors and morbidity. Ophthalmology. 2006;113:109.

42. Wagner H, Richdale K, Mitchell GL, et al. Age, behavior, environment, and health factors in the soft contact lens risk survey. Optom Vis Sci. 2014;91:252.

43. Liesegang TJ. Herpes simplex virus epidemiology and ocular importance. Cornea. 2001;20(1):1–13.

44. Souza PM, Holland EJ, Huang AJ. Bilateral herpetic keratoconjunctivitis. Ophthalmology. 2003;110:493.

45. Oral acyclovir for herpes simplex virus eye disease: effect on prevention of epithelial keratitis and stromal keratitis. Herpetic eye disease study group. Arch Ophthalmol. 2000;118:1030.

46. Gonzalez-Gonzalez LA, Molina-Prat N, Doctor P, et al. Clinical features and presentation of infectious scleritis from herpes viruses: a report of 35 cases. Ophthalmology. 2012;119:1460.

47. Vrcek I, Choudhury E, Durairaj V. Herpes zoster ophthalmicus: a review for the internist. Am J Med. 2016;130(1):21–6. https://doi.org/10.1016/j.amjmed.2016.08.039.

48. Keenan JD, Mcleod SD. 4.12 – Bacterial keratitis. 4th ed. Amsterdam: Elsevier; 2016. https://doi.org/10.1016/B978-1-4557-3984-4.00121-4.

49. Smolin G, Foster CS, Azar DT, Dohlman CH. Smolin and Thoft's the cornea: scientific foundations and clinical practice. Philadelphia, PA: Lippincott Williams & Wilkins; 2005.

50. Bennett JE, Dolin R, Blaser MJ. Microbial keratitis. In: Mandell, Douglas, and Bennett's principles and practice of infectious diseases. Philadelphia: Elsevier Health Sciences; 2014.

51. Yanoff M, Jay S. Bacterial keratitis. In: Duker, editor. Ophthalmology; 2014.

52. Yanoff M, Jay S. Fungal keratitis. In: Duker, editor. Ophthalmology; 2014.

53. Acharya NR, Tham VM, Esterberg E, et al. Incidence and prevalence of uveitis. JAMA Ophthalmol. 2013;131(11):1405. https://doi.org/10.1001/jamaophthalmol.2013.4237.

54. Read R. General approach to the uveitis patient and treatment strategies. In: Yanoff M, editor. Ophthalmology. 4th ed. Amsterdam: Elsevier; 2014. p. 694–9.

55. McCannel CA, Holland GN, Helm CJ, et al. Causes of uveitis in the general practice of ophthalmology. Am J Ophthalmol. 1996;121(1):35–46. https://doi.org/10.1016/S0002-9394(14)70532-X.

56. Bennett JE, Dolin R, Blaser MJ. Endophthalmitis. In: Mandell, Douglas, and Bennett's principles and practice of infectious diseases. Philadelphia: Elsevier Health Sciences; 2014.

57. Endophthalmitis Vitrectomy Study Group. Results of the Endophthalmitis Vitrectomy study. A randomized trial of immediate vitrectomy and of intravenous antibiotics for the treatment of postoperative bacterial endophthalmitis. Arch Ophthalmol. 1995;113:1479–96.

58. Klotz SA, Penn CC, Negvesky GJ, Butrus SI. Fungal and parasitic infections of the eye. Clin Microbiol Rev. 2000;13(4):662–85.

59. Kanski JJ, Bowling B. Clinical ophthalmology: a systemic approach. 7th ed. New York: Elsevier Saunders; 2011. p. 34–9.

60. Lopez Montero, Martha Cecilia. Conjunctivitis. http://eyewiki.aao.org/Conjunctivitis - accessed 29 May 2017.

61. US Food and Drug Administration. FDA News Release: FDA approves besivance to treat bacterial conjunctivitis. May 28, 2009.

62. Garg P, Rao GN. Corneal ulcer: diagnosis and management. Community Eye Health. 1999;12(30):21–3.

63. Wilhelmus KR. Antiviral treatment and other therapeutic interventions for herpes simplex virus epithelial keratitis. Cochrane Database Syst Rev. 2015;1:CD002898.

64. Collum LM, McGettrick P, Akhtar J, et al. Oral acyclovir (Zovirax) in herpes simplex dendritic corneal ulceration. Br J Ophthalmol. 1986;70:435.

65. Colin J, Hoh HB, Easty DL, et al. Ganciclovir ophthalmic gel (Virgan; 0.15%) in the treatment of herpes simplex keratitis. Cornea. 1997;16:393.

66. A controlled trial of oral acyclovir for the prevention of stromal keratitis or iritis in patients with herpes simplex virus epithelial keratitis. The epithelial keratitis trial. The Herpetic Eye Disease Study Group. Arch Ophthalmol. 1997;115:703.

67. Keenan JD, Mcleod SD. 4.13 – Fungal keratitis. 4th ed. Amsterdam: Elsevier; 2016. https://doi.org/10.1016/B978-1-4557-3984-4.00122-6.

68. Thomas PA. Fungal infections of the cornea. Eye (Lond). 2003;17(8):852–62. https://doi.org/10.1038/sj.eye.6700557.

69. Jurkunas U, Behlau I, Colby K. Fungal keratitis: changing pathogens and risk factors. Cornea. 2009;28(6):638–43. https://doi.org/10.1097/ICO.0b013e318191695b.

70. Chern KC. Emergency ophthalmology: a rapid treatment guide. New York: McGraw-Hill Professional; 2002.

Chapter 11
Neuro-ophthalmologic Emergencies

James L. Webb and Brit Long

Brief Introduction

Neuro-ophthalmologic emergencies consist of neurologic disorders that have ocular involvement. These conditions often require urgent imaging, consultation, and treatment. The ophthalmologic presentation along with associated features can guide the emergency physician in localizing the underlying process and subsequent management.

Clinical Presentation

Various ophthalmologic complaints can be a presenting symptom with a neurologic etiology.

Such symptoms include vision loss, diplopia, pupillary defect, ophthalmoplegias, papilledema, or nystagmus. Particular

J. L. Webb, MD
San Antonio Uniformed Services Health Education Consortium, San Antonio, TX, USA

B. Long, MD (✉)
San Antonio Military Medical Center, Department of Emergency Medicine, San Antonio, TX, USA

© Springer International Publishing AG, part of Springer Nature 2018
B. Long, A. Koyfman (eds.), *Handbook of Emergency Ophthalmology*, https://doi.org/10.1007/978-3-319-78945-3_11

neurologic disorders should be considered according to the ocular symptoms with consideration of the patient's comorbidities, associated symptoms, and level of consciousness. For neuro-ophthalmologic disorders, an understanding of the neuroanatomy in relation to the ocular symptoms is crucial.

Differential Diagnosis

Neurologic sources of vision loss include cerebral infarct or hemorrhage, neoplasm, giant cell arteritis, optic neuritis, parasellar mass, migraine headaches, and idiopathic intracranial hypertension. Other, non-neurologic sources include amaurosis fugax, central retinal artery occlusion, central retinal vein occlusion, glaucoma, trauma, keratitis, uveitis, hyphema, retinal detachment, vitreous hemorrhage, cataracts, macular degeneration, lens pathologies, and functional blindness. Visual field defects include any lesion along the optic pathway from the optic nerve to the occipital lobe. This includes cerebral ischemia or hemorrhage, trauma, neoplasm, vasculitis, infection, and retinal detachment. The differential for neurologic source of diplopia includes cranial nerve palsies, posterior communicating artery aneurysm, and myasthenia gravis. Other sources of diplopia include extraocular muscle obstruction (thyroid ophthalmopathy or muscle entrapment) and autoimmune and vascular pathologies. The differential for pupil asymmetry includes physiologic, history of trauma or surgery, third nerve compression (hemorrhage or neoplasm), uncal herniation, intracranial mass (hematoma, neoplasm, or edema due to stroke), or topical medications such as anticholinergics. The differential for papilledema includes malignant hypertension, intracranial masses (hematoma or tumor), cerebral edema, idiopathic intracranial hypertension, and hydrocephalus. Related vascular disorders should be kept in mind when considering neuro-ophthalmologic disorders including posterior communicating artery aneurysm, carotid artery dissection, cavernous sinus syndrome, and pituitary apoplexy.

Other focal neurologic deficits should be considered when approaching the differential. The level of consciousness can help narrow the etiology and dictate urgency in care. Important features that should also be considered include painful vision loss, afferent pupillary defect, and abnormal funduscopic exam.

Clinical Evaluation

History

A detailed history of the ocular complaints and associated symptoms is essential. Symptoms that should be considered are vision loss, visual field deficits, blurred vision, diplopia, ptosis, and pupil asymmetry [1, 2].

- If there is vision loss, it should be characterized by painful or painless, one or both eyes, timing of onset, and degree and area of vision loss.
- If there is diplopia, ask if it is worse or better by any gaze position.
- If there is ptosis, determine if it is unilateral or worse at different times of the day.
- If the pupils are asymmetric, ask if it is chronic or new to the patient.
- Other ophthalmic complaints such as redness or discharge.
- Determine if trauma was involved.
- Determine if there is a difference in color vision, particularly red desaturation, which can be seen in optic nerve disease.
- Associated symptoms to pay attention include headache, nausea, vomiting, neck pain, and other focal neuro deficits.

Past Medical History

The past medical history includes vascular disease (hypertension, diabetes, hypercoagulability), stroke history, history of prior vision loss or neuro deficits, use of contact lenses, history of eye surgery, and topical or ophthalmic medication use (such as scopolamine patches). Previous surgeries can cause irregular pupil size. History of hypertension and diabetes can result in ischemic cranial nerve palsies [1, 2].

Physical Exam

After the history, a thorough physical exam can narrow down the etiology. The patient's level of consciousness should direct the urgency of care. Performing an exam sequentially can help avoid missing a key piece of information. The following should be tested in the ophthalmologic exam [1, 2].

1. *General inspection*: determine the level of consciousness and evaluate the eyelids and sclera, observing for ptosis or proptosis.
2. *Visual acuity*: this should be done based on a Snellen eye chart. Each eye should be examined separately.
   - Test should be done with the patient's glasses or contact lenses. If the patient does not have these available, a pinhole can be used for correction.
   - If unable to see the letters, finger counting, and hand motions, or if still having difficulty, light perception can be used.
   - Observe for difference in color perception, particularly red desaturation.
   - If the patient claims to have blindness with an otherwise normal exam, evaluate for functional blindness. One method is the mirror test: rotating a mirror in front of a patient to observe for tracking.
3. *Visual fields*: evaluate all four quadrants by either hand movement or number of fingers in the peripheral vision field.
4. *Pupils*: evaluate the size, symmetry, and reactivity to light.
5. *Extraocular movements*: cranial nerves III, IV, and VI.
6. Apply *fluorescein* if there is concern for abrasions or ulcer.

7. Test *intraocular pressure* by tonometry. Normal pressure is 10–20 mmHg.
8. *Funduscopic exam*: Inspect the posterior chamber preferably with dilation. Note the optic disk and vasculature. Observe for papilledema.
9. Use the *slit lamp* if there is concern for anterior chamber pathology.
10. *Ocular US* can assist in evaluating the optic nerve, as well as the vitreous.

Clinical Conditions and Management

Vision Loss

Vision loss can be due to a process in the globe itself or a neurologic cause, which can be difficult to differentiate. Vision starts with light entering the pupil, which is converted to neuronal impulses at the retina and transmitted along the optic pathway to the occipital cortex. A disruption anywhere in this conduction causes vision loss. Disorders of the globe include media abnormalities and retinal detachment. Retinal vascular disease (central retinal artery occlusion or central retinal vein occlusion) may mimic optic neuropathies with optic disk swelling and vision loss. The optic pathways include the optic nerves, which cross at the optic chiasm, the optic tract, the optic radiations, and the occipital cortex. Characteristics of vision loss that can narrow the differential down include painless or painful, how rapid the onset is, degree and area of visual field deficit, presence of an afferent pupillary defect, funduscopic exam, and history and physical exam. On physical exam, improvement with pinhole suggests a non-neurologic source [1–3].

Visual Field Deficits

The areas of visual field deficits can help localize the lesion and narrow the etiology. A defect can be caused by a lesion anywhere along the optic pathway (Fig. 11.1). Optic neuritis

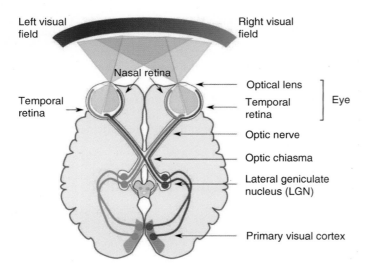

FIGURE. 11.1 Representation of the visual pathway with examples of lesions. Image from https://upload.wikimedia.org/wikipedia/commons/thumb/b/bf/Human_visual_pathway.svg/1000px-Human_visual_pathway.svg.png

can present as monocular complete vision loss with an afferent pupillary defect. Rapid, monocular vision loss is often due to a vascular source such as central retinal artery occlusion. Compression of the optic chiasm often presents as bitemporal hemianopia (visual loss of the temporal halves). Homonymous hemianopia (visual loss of both left halves and right halves) is seen in optic tract lesions. Homonymous quadrantanopia (visual loss of one quadrant bilaterally) is seen in optic radiation lesions (superior quadrantanopia in temporal radiations and inferior quadrantanopia in parietal radiations). Occipital lobe lesions result in homonymous hemianopia. In ischemic occipital lobe lesions, central (macula) vision may be spared due to dual blood supply of the occipital poles [2–5].

Homonymous hemianopia is often caused by cerebral infarction or hemorrhage. Specifically, causes of optic nerve lesion include inflammatory processes, vasculitis, ischemia, infections, and neoplasm. Lesions of the optic chiasm are commonly due to a parasellar mass (such as pituitary adenoma). Optic tract and optic radiation lesions include neoplasm, ischemia, inflammation, and infections. Occipital lobe lesions are due to similar pathologies, ischemia being the most common. Visual field defects require neuroimaging, and neurology should be consulted [2–5].

Giant Cell Arteritis

Giant cell arteritis or temporal arteritis is a systemic vasculitis of medium- and large-sized arteries that can cause anterior ischemic optic neuropathy and, less frequently, central retinal artery occlusion. Typically it presents as a painless, gradual onset vision loss with an afferent pupillary defect. Patients are rarely younger than 50. It is often seen in Caucasian females and associated with a history of polymyalgia rheumatica. Presenting symptoms include headache (in 90% of patients), jaw claudication, fever, fatigue, myalgias, weight loss, and temporal artery tenderness. ESR and CRP are usually elevated. Funduscopic exam shows a chalky white optic disk. A temporal artery biopsy is needed for definitive diagnosis, but a negative biopsy does not exclude it. Treat with methylprednisolone 1 g IV if patient has visual symptoms. Treatment should not be delayed for obtaining the biopsy. Vision loss is usually permanent, and contralateral ocular involvement often occurs in days to weeks without treatment [1–4, 6, 7].

Optic Nerve Ischemia

Ischemic optic neuropathy is due to vascular insufficiency causing hypoperfusion and ischemia. It is more common in elderly patients. It can be seen in small-vessel disease of the anterior optic nerve. It is acute, monocular, and painless. Optic disk swelling will be noted on funduscopic exam if the anterior portion is involved. Vasculitides, primarily giant cell arteritis, are the most common cause of anterior and posterior ischemic optic neuritis [4, 8].

Optic Neuritis

Optic neuritis can be caused by infection (viral infection, syphilis, tuberculosis, or cryptococcus), inflammatory disease (sarcoidosis), and commonly due to demyelination. Acute demyelinating optic neuritis is highly associated with multiple sclerosis. Patients are often young females. Vision loss is typically monocular and painful (particularly with eye movements) and occurs over hours to days and with an afferent pupil defect. Color vision is more commonly affected than acuity, where a red object will appear lighter in the affected eye. Funduscopic exam is often normal but may show an edematous optic disk. An MRI of the head should be obtained to evaluate for optic white matter lesions to confirm the diagnosis. An MRI is also useful to evaluate brain white matter changes to assess the risk of developing MS. Treatment involves methylprednisolone 1 g IV for 3 days followed by an oral prednisone taper. Ophthalmology and neurology should be consulted for further workup and follow-up [1–4, 9–11].

Stroke/Cortical Blindness

Cerebral ischemia can present with ophthalmologic defects depending on the location. If ischemia occurs in the anterior circulation, it can result with monocular blindness. Occipital lobe ischemia or infarction, located in the posterior circulation, can result in bilateral vision loss or visual field deficits (cortical blindness). Large areas of ischemia can show eye deviation ipsilateral to the insult. Associated neurologic deficits are often seen which help localize the lesion. Diagnosis includes prompt imaging with CT/CTA, MRI/MRA, and neurology consult [1–4].

Floaters/Flashing Lights

Floaters can be a benign process. Idiopathic vitreous floaters are a common cause. However, acute monocular flashing lights or floaters are usually due to a process within the globe such as retinal detachment/tear or vitreous detachment. Patients with monocular floaters with vision loss should be seen by an ophthalmologist urgently for potential retinal surgery. If it is binocular, it is usually due to a neurologic source, commonly migraines which are associated with headache, nausea, and vomiting. The visual aura often begins laterally and develops a shimmering or flashing quality. Migraines with aura are sudden onset with a normal funduscopic exam. Monocular retinal migraines are rare and present as a reoccurring headache with monocular scotomata that lasts less than an hour [1, 12–14].

Functional Vision Loss

Functional vision loss is due to a nonanatomical source, such as conversion disorder or malingering. Vision loss is painless, can range from sudden onset to gradual, and has a normal funduscopic exam. Symptoms are inconsistent with neurologic pathology. Some physical exam findings associated with functional vision loss include resistance to eye opening or geotropic gaze on head turning. One maneuver to evaluate is the mirror test: rotating a mirror in front of the patient and observing for pursuit. Those due to conversion disorder are true blindness, and frequently patients are indifferent about the symptoms. Other visual symptoms include blurred vision, diplopia, and nystagmus. It is a diagnosis of exclusion, and treatment is tailored to the underline psychiatric disorder [1, 2, 15, 16].

Diplopia

Diplopia is seeing two images of a single object. Monocular diplopia is often due to a process within the globe such as cataracts, lens pathologies or corneal irregularity, and rarely from a neurologic source. Resolution of diplopia when covering either eye suggests a problem with the extraocular muscles or their innervation. The most common cause of binocular diplopia is cranial nerve palsy due to microvascular disease. Cranial nerve palsies result in misalignment in specific gaze positions. There are six cardinal directions controlled by the six extraocular muscles which are innervated by the third, fourth, and sixth cranial nerves. Isolated cranial nerve palsy can be self-limiting, but if there are associated neurologic symptoms, it raises concern for a more emergent etiology such as stroke, intracranial masses, aneurysm, infection, or trauma. Associate red flags include pain (headache or neck pain), papilledema, pupil asymmetry, nystagmus, or visual field deficits. Inability to manually move the eye is suggestive of a restrictive process such as thyroid disease or muscle entrapment. Neuromuscular junction disorders (myasthenia gravis) can also affect eye movement. Cranial nerve palsies are discussed below [1–4].

CN III Palsy

CN III innervates the extraocular muscles for adduction, elevation, and depression and the levator muscle of the eyelid. It also controls pupil constriction through the efferent parasympathetic fibers. Injury to these fibers results in pupillary dilation. Chronic third nerve palsy is often due to microvascular disease from diabetes and hypertension resulting in infarction of the central nerve fibers. A complete palsy will present with diplopia, ptosis, pupil dilation, and a down and outward positioned eye, though they are often incomplete. In third nerve palsy due to microvascular disease, the pupillary reflex frequently remains intact since the parasympathetic fibers run on the periphery which is less affected. Symptoms beyond an isolated third nerve (altered mental status, other cranial nerve involvement, recent trauma) should raise concern for other etiologies. These include processes involving the subarachnoid space —inflammation, infection, or malignancies of the meninges. Others include uncal herniation, cavernous-carotid fistula, or myasthenia gravis. In patients with isolated pupil-sparing third nerve palsy with high suspicion of ischemic injury and vascular risk factors, observation and follow-up are appropriate. However, further workup should be considered if suspicious of aneurysm or other etiology [1–4, 17].

Posterior Communicating Artery Aneurysm

Third nerve palsy with a dilated and unreactive pupil should raise concern for an intracranial aneurysm. The peripheral parasympathetic fibers are more susceptible to compression resulting in unresponsive pupillary dilation. The most common source is the posterior communicating artery which causes compression on the cranial nerve. An enlarging aneurysm causing third nerve palsy is at risk of rupture and is life-threatening. Therefore, if an aneurysm is suspected, urgent neuroimaging is necessary. Treatment includes blood pressure control and neurosurgery consult [1–3, 18].

CN IV Palsy

CN IV innervates the superior oblique muscle which controls depression and intorsion. A patient with fourth nerve palsy presents with vertical diplopia and may turn the head to compensate. The most common cause is due to trauma, but microvascular disease can cause dysfunction as well [2, 4].

CN VI Palsy

CN VI controls the lateral rectus muscle for abduction. Sixth nerve palsy results in lateral gaze defect and horizontal diplopia. Diplopia is worse upon ipsilateral eye abduction, and patients can present with inward deviation. Sixth nerve palsy can be caused by microvascular disease similar to the other cranial nerve palsies. However, given its long course, the sixth nerve is vulnerable to trauma, tumors, or increased intracranial pressure compression. Bilateral sixth nerve palsy, multiple cranial nerve involvement, or associated papilledema are red flags for increased intracranial pressure or neoplasm. Associated symptoms of headache, nausea, or fever are suggestive of an infectious etiology. Thyroid disease involving the medial rectus muscle can cause movement restriction and present similarly to sixth nerve palsy. Neuroimaging is necessary to rule out an intracranial lesion, but if other etiologies are excluded, isolated sixth nerve palsy can be observed with follow-up [1, 2, 4].

Vascular Lesions

The blood supply of the orbit is from the ophthalmic artery, which is a branch of the internal carotid artery. The central retinal artery comes off the ophthalmic artery. The central retinal vein drains the orbit which communicates with the cavernous sinus. The sympathetic fibers responsible for pupil dilation start in the hypothalamus and have second-order neurons that exit the spinal cord and run along the sympathetic chain to the superior cervical ganglion and third-order neurons that travel along the carotid artery to the orbit. Injury to any of these fibers results in miosis [1–4].

Horner Syndrome/Carotid Artery Dissection

The classic triad of Horner syndrome is miosis, ptosis, and anhidrosis. It is caused by a lesion in the sympathetic pathway to the neck, head, and eye. Ptosis is usually milder than in third nerve palsy, and anhidrosis may not be present depending on the location of the lesion. An internal carotid artery dissection can cause Horner syndrome, and patients may present with neck pain or with a history of trauma. Other etiologies include stroke and neoplasm which usually present with other associated symptoms such as weakness, ataxia, or vertigo. Workup includes chest X-ray, CT of the head and cervical region, and CTA or MRA of the head and neck to evaluate for carotid dissection [1, 2, 4, 19].

Cavernous Sinus Syndrome

Cranial nerves III, IV, V1, V2, and VI, along with the carotid artery, run through the cavernous sinus located lateral to the pituitary fossa and posterior to the orbit. A lesion in this area can cause a syndrome of orbital pain, ophthalmoplegias, ptosis, and V1 and V2 numbness. However, isolated third or sixth nerve palsies may be present in partial syndromes. Etiologies include primary neoplasm, metastases, carotid aneurysm, carotid-cavernous fistula, and septic thrombosis. A carotid-cavernous fistula secondary to intracavernous carotid artery rupture presents with pulsating proptosis, ocular bruits, and conjunctival chemosis and is life-threatening. Septic thrombosis is often secondary to sinus, facial, or dental infection and can present with headache, fever, and chemosis. The most common pathogen is *Staphylococcus aureus* and less frequently streptococci. Diagnosis involves urgent neuroimaging and treatment of a fistula (surgical/endovascular intervention) or thrombosis (prompt empiric antimicrobial therapy and often anticoagulation) [2, 4, 20, 21].

Pituitary Apoplexy

Lesions at the optic chiasm can be caused by compression from a pituitary tumor or hemorrhage. Pituitary apoplexy is the hemorrhagic infarction of the pituitary gland often secondary to a previous pituitary lesion. Patients present with sudden onset severe headache, visual field defects (often bitemporal hemianopia), and decreased visual acuity. Endocrine changes (hypopituitarism) may also occur. Workup includes neuroimaging (MRI can detect hemorrhage more frequently than CT) and neurosurgery consult for potential surgical decompression, which is often indicated if visual symptoms are involved [4, 22–24].

Increased Intracranial Pressure/Papilledema

Papilledema is caused by increased intracranial pressure (ICP) leading to optic disk swelling on funduscopic exam (Fig. 11.2). Optic disk swelling (not caused by increase ICP) can also be seen in infectious and inflammatory disorders such as syphilis, HIV, and lupus. Associated symptoms of increased ICP include headache, nausea, vomiting, diplopia, and other neurologic

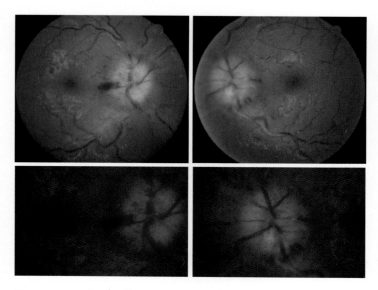

FIGURE. 11.2 Optic disk with moderate papilledema. Image from https://webeye.ophth.uiowa.edu/eyeforum/atlas/pages/papilledema-secondary-to-meningitis/index.htm

deficits. The differential of increased ICP includes intracranial mass, idiopathic intracranial hypertension (pseudotumor cerebri), cerebral edema, cerebral venous thrombosis, and hydrocephalus. CN VI is susceptible to increased ICP, and unilateral or bilateral sixth nerve palsy can be present. Bedside ultrasound can be useful in detecting optic disk edema, with optic nerve sheath diameter greater than 5 mm. Papilledema requires immediate neuroimaging and LP if there is an absence of a mass that could lead to herniation [1–4].

Idiopathic Intracranial Hypertension (Pseudotumor Cerebri)

Idiopathic intracranial hypertension is due to increased ICP and presents with normal CSF cell studies and normal neuroimaging. Opening pressure is typically elevated. Patients present with headache, nausea, vomiting, transient blurred vision, and papilledema. Visual field deficits may be present. It is associated with female gender, obesity, and certain medications (glucocorticoids, vitamin A, and tetracyclines). Workup includes neuroimaging (either CT or MRI) followed by an LP with opening pressure and routine CSF laboratories to rule out other etiologies. Treatment is with acetazolamide and weight loss. Other diuretics and carbonic anhydrase inhibitors can be used if symptoms do not improve. Severe or progressive vision loss may require hospitalization for surgical intervention such as a shunt [1, 4, 25, 26].

Myasthenia Gravis

In myasthenia gravis, patients present with intermittent diplopia and/or ptosis due to the extraocular muscle fatigue caused by a neuromuscular junction disorder. It may only involve ocular symptoms or have a generalized presentation involving oculomotor, extremity, and respiratory muscle fatigue. Apart from diplopia and ptosis, which are the most common symptoms, patients may have dysarthria, dysphagia, chewing fatigue, extremity weakness, or respiratory insufficiency (ranging from exertional dyspnea to respiratory failure). Symptoms are often worse with activity, later in the day, and can be provoked with prolonged or repetitive movements. Age of onset is bimodal: occurring early (before 40; often in females) or late (after 60; often in males). Diagnosis can be supported with fatigability on sustained upward gaze or the ice pack test (improvement in ptosis after placing an ice pack on the eyelid for 2 min). If suspected, the patient will need a neurology consult and definitive diagnosis with laboratory testing [2, 3, 27, 28].

Wernicke's Encephalopathy

Nutritional deficits can present with oculomotor abnormalities. Wernicke's encephalopathy is due to a thiamine deficiency and can present with a triad of altered mental status, ataxia, and oculomotor abnormalities. The presenting ocular finding is commonly nystagmus, but others can be seen such as sixth never palsy, pupil asymmetry, retinal hemorrhage, or ptosis. It is most commonly associated with chronic alcoholism but is seen in other sources of malnutrition or malabsorption. Diagnosis is primarily clinical. Neuroimaging may contribute, but it should not delay treatment. Treatment is with prompt IV thiamine 500 mg [2, 4, 29, 30].

Disposition

The emergency physician is frequently responsible for the urgent assessment of neuro-ophthalmic disorders. Urgent neuroimaging should be performed for concern of visual field defects caused by ischemia or hemorrhage, stroke, posterior communicating artery aneurysm, CN VI palsy, carotid artery dissection, cavernous sinus syndrome, pituitary apoplexy, or papilledema. Neuroimaging is part of the workup of optic neuritis, other cranial nerve palsies, and Horner syndrome. Urgent consults (to neurology and/or ophthalmology) are required for visual field defects suspicious of an intracranial lesion, optic neuritis, stroke, and myasthenia gravis. Consult neurosurgery regarding posterior communicating artery aneurysm, cavernous sinus syndrome due to fistula, and pituitary apoplexy. Urgent treatment is necessary for giant cell arteritis, optic neuritis, cavernous sinus thrombosis, and Wernicke's encephalopathy.

Pearls/Pitfalls

Neurologic disorders can present with ophthalmologic symptoms and often require prompt evaluation, imaging, and treatment.

1. History including specific ophthalmologic symptom, degree of vision loss, presence of ptosis or pupil asymmetry, and any associated symptoms or focal neurologic deficits.

2. Physical exam including general inspection, visual acuity, visual fields, pupils, extraocular movements, fluorescein, intraocular pressure, funduscopic exam, slit lamp, and ultrasound.

3. Urgent neuroimaging is needed for concern of visual field defects caused by ischemia or hemorrhage, stroke, posterior communicating artery aneurysm, CN VI palsy, carotid artery dissection, cavernous sinus syndrome, pituitary apoplexy, or papilledema.

4. Urgent consultation (to neurology and/or ophthalmology) should be made for visual field defects suspicious of an intracranial lesion, optic neuritis, stroke, and myasthenia gravis. Neurosurgery should be consulted for posterior communicating artery aneurysm, cavernous sinus syndrome due to fistula, and pituitary apoplexy.

5. Urgent treatment is required for giant cell arteritis, optic neuritis, cavernous sinus thrombosis, and Wernicke's encephalopathy.

References

1. Walker RA, Adhikaris. Eye emergencies. In: Tintinalli's emergency medicine: a comprehensive study guide. 8th ed. Columbus: Mcgraw-Hill; 2016. Chap. 241.

2. Huff JS, Austin EW. Neuro-ophthalmology in emergency medicine. Emerg Med Clin North Am. 2016;34:967–86.

3. Cordonnier M, Van Nechel C. Neuro-ophthalmological emergencies: which ocular signs or symptoms for which diseases? Acta Neurol Belg. 2013;113:215–24.

4. Graves JS, Galetta SL. Acute visual loss and other neuro-ophthalmologic emergencies: management. Neurol Clin. 2012;30:75–99.

5. Zhang X, Kedar S, Lynn MJ, et al. Homonymous hemianopias: clinical-anatomic correlations in 904 cases. Neurology. 2006;66:906.

6. Kawasaki A, Purvin V. Giant cell arteritis: an updated review. Acta Ophthalmol. 2009;87:13–32.

7. Smetana GW, Shmerling RH. Does this patient have temporal arteritis? JAMA. 2002;287:92–101.

8. Biousse V, Newman NJ. Ischemic optic neuropathies. N Engl J Med. 2015;372:2428–36.

9. Balcer LJ. Clinical practice. Optic neuritis. N Engl J Med. 2006;354:1273–80.

10. Arnold AC. Evolving management of optic neuritis and multiple sclerosis. Am J Ophthalmol. 2005;139:1101–8.

11. Golnik KC. Infectious optic neuropathy. Semin Ophthalmol. 2002;17:11–7.

12. Hollands H, Johnson D, Brox AC, et al. Acute-onset floaters and flashes: is this patient at risk for retinal detachment? JAMA. 2009;302:2243–9.

13. Charles A. Advances in the basic and clinical science of migraine. Ann Neurol. 2009;65:491–8.

14. Cutrer FM, Huerter K. Migraine aura. Neurologist. 2007;13:118–25.

15. Stone J, Carson A, Sharpe M. Functional symptoms and signs in neurology: assessment and diagnosis. J Neurol Neurosurg Psychiatry. 2005;76(Suppl 1):i2–12.

16. Beatty S. Non-organic visual loss. Postgrad Med J. 1999;75:201–7.

17. Lee SH, Lee SS, Park KY, Han SH. Isolated oculomotor nerve palsy: diagnostic approach using the degree of external and internal dysfunction. Clin Neurol Neurosurg. 2002;104:136.

18. Chaudhary N, Davagnanam I, Ansari SA, et al. Imaging of intracranial aneurysms causing isolated third cranial nerve palsy. J Neuroophthalmol. 2009;29:238–44.

19. Walton KA, Buono LM. Horner syndrome. Curr Opin Ophthalmol. 2003;14:357–63.

20. Bone I, Hadley DM. Syndromes of the orbital fissure, cavernous sinus, cerebello-pontine angle, and skull base. J Neurol Neurosurg Psychiatry. 2005;76(Suppl 3):iii29–38.

21. Ebright JR, Pace MT, Niazi AF. Septic thrombosis of the cavernous sinuses. Arch Intern Med. 2001;161:2671–6.

22. Randeva HS, Schoebel J, Byrne J, et al. Classical pituitary apoplexy: clinical features, management and outcome. Clin Endocrinol. 1999;51:181–8.

23. Capatina C, Inder W, Karavitaki N, Wass JA. Management of endocrine disease: pituitary tumour apoplexy. Eur J Endocrinol. 2015;172:R179–90.

24. Arafah BM, Harrington JF, Madhoun ZT, Selman WR. Improvement of pituitary function after surgical decompression for pituitary tumor apoplexy. J Clin Endocrinol Metab. 1990;71:323–8.

25. Wall M, Kupersmith MJ, Kieburtz KD, et al. The idiopathic intra-cranial hypertension treatment trial: clinical profile at baseline. JAMA Neurol. 2014;71:693–701.

26. Biousse V, Bruce BB, Newman NJ. Update on the pathophysiol-ogy and management of idiopathic intracranial hypertension. J Neurol Neurosurg Psychiatry. 2012;83:488–94.

27. Silvestri NJ, Wolfe GI. Myasthenia gravis. Semin Neurol. 2012;32:215–26.

28. Meriggioli MN, Sanders DB. Autoimmune myasthenia gravis: emerging clinical and biological heterogeneity. Lancet Neurol. 2009;8:475.

29. Donnino MW, Vega J, Miller J, Walsh M. Myths and miscon-ceptions of Wernicke's encephalopathy: what every emergency physician should know. Ann Emerg Med. 2007;50:715–21.

30. Galvin R, Bråthen G, Ivashynka A, et al. EFNS guidelines for diagnosis, therapy and prevention of Wernicke encephalopathy. Eur J Neurol. 2010;17:1408–18.

Chapter 12
Ocular Burns and Exposures

Daniel Reschke

Brief Introduction

Ocular chemical, thermal, and radiation burns represent a significant proportion of ocular trauma presenting to the emergency department [1, 2]. Exposures to bodily fluids and cyanoacrylates (super glues) also carry important clinical implications. Without proper evaluation and prompt treatment by the emergency physician, ocular burns and exposures can be a source of intense pain and potential vision loss.

Clinical Presentation

Patients with chemical burns often present with pain after a known exposure to a chemical. Exposures from gas, liquids, solids, and powders may cause damage. Chemical burns are caused by a wide array of substances ranging from industrial chemicals to children's party bubbles [3, 4]. Common offending agents include household cleaning products, cosmetics, anti-personal sprays, and industrial material [4–6].

D. Reschke, MD
Emergency Medicine, San Antonio Uniformed Services Health Education Consortium, San Antonio, TX, USA

© Springer International Publishing AG, part of Springer Nature 2018
B. Long, A. Koyfman (eds.), *Handbook of Emergency Ophthalmology*, https://doi.org/10.1007/978-3-319-78945-3_12

211

Some exposures are less obvious, such as those from airbag deployment following MVC, and require a high index of suspicion [7]. Thermal burns are rare due to a rapid lid reflex but may occur with exposure to hot liquids, direct flame, and fireworks. Radiation burns arise from prolonged unprotected exposure to UV light, often indirectly from snow (i.e., snow blindness) or directly (i.e., tanning beds, welders arcs, and solar eclipse viewing) [4, 6]. Ocular exposure to bodily fluids will most likely occur in the healthcare setting and raises concern for acquisition of infectious disease. Ocular cyanoacrylate exposure occurs in the home (i.e., when glue bottles are mistaken for eye drops) or is iatrogenic in nature (i.e., during laceration repair) [8–10].

Clinical Evaluation

History

The history for an ocular exposure is key in directing initial treatment and determining prognosis. For each exposure, there are several important elements of the history to obtain:

- Determine the causative agent resulting in the exposure. For chemicals, determine if the chemical is alkaline or acidic in nature (see Table 12.1).
- Determine the amount of material exposed to the eye.
- Determine the length of exposure.
- Assess level of pain.

For bodily fluid exposures, obtain the following [11]:

- The date/time and fluid type involved.
- From the source patient, obtain the following: hepatitis B, hepatitis C, and HIV status. Also obtain information regarding the following risk factors: high-risk sexual practices, IV drug use, hemophilia, and transfusion history.
- From the exposed patient, obtain the following: last tetanus, HBV vaccination, and pregnancy status.

TABLE 12.1 Chemical composition and pH properties of common commercial products

Commercial product	Chemical
Alkalis	
Cement Lime Plaster	Calcium hydroxide
Cement Lime	Calcium carbonate
Drain cleaner Oven cleaner Lye	Sodium hydroxide
Ammonia (cleaner/fertilizer)	Ammonium hydroxide
Bleach	Sodium hypochlorite
Laundry detergent	Sodium carbonate
Acids	
Toilet cleaner	Sulfuric acid/hydrochloric acid
Rust remover Glass etching/metal working High octane gasoline	Hydrofluoric acid
Car battery	Sulfuric acid

Physical Exam

Ocular exposures are unique because the majority of the physical exam will follow initial treatment measures. After copious irrigation, perform the following:

- Assess visual acuity, IOP, pupillary size and reaction, and extra ocular movements.
- Inspect the cornea, conjunctiva, and surrounding structures. Common findings include epiphora (tearing), conjunctival chemosis, and injection. The cornea should be carefully examined for haze or opacification. It is critical to note the presence or absence of limbal, conjunctival,

or scleral whitening, which indicates ischemia. At first glance, a "white and quiet" eye can mistakenly be documented as normal, while paradoxically the blanched vessels and ischemia are indicators of severe injury and poor prognosis.

- Be sure to have the patient look in all directions, inspect the conjunctival fornices, and evert the eyelids. Remove residual particulate matter with a moist cotton swab under topical anesthesia with proparacaine.
- Perform a detailed slit lamp exam with fluorescein, being careful to note the extent of corneal or conjunctival epithelial defects.
- Assess for lagophthalmos (inability to fully close the eyelid).
- Ocular burns are classically classified by the Roper-Hall system based on the amount of corneal damage and limbal evolvement. Recently, the Dua system has suggested focusing purely on limbal involvement evolvement. A complete opacification and loss of vascularization at the limbus indicates limbal ischemia. This is associated with more severe injury and a poor prognosis, as the stem cells that regenerate the corneal epithelium reside at the limbus [12, 13].

Clinical Conditions

1. *Ocular burns*

   (a) *Chemical burns* primarily result in corneal and scleral damage. Alkaline substances are typically lipophilic and result in liquefactive necrosis, allowing the chemical to penetrate deep into tissue, causing more extensive damage than acids. Irreversible damage occurs with a pH higher than 11.5 [14]. Acids result in coagulation necrosis, forming a barrier that prevents further penetration of the chemical. Hydrofluoric acid (HF) is a particularly damaging acid. HF does not readily dissociate and can penetrate deep into the tissues.

HF also has important treatment considerations that differ from those of other acids [15].

(b) *Thermal burns* to the globe itself are rare and more commonly affect the eyelid and surrounding adnexal structures. In one study, only 15% of patients with facial burns had injury to the ocular globe or eyelid. Serious ocular pathology and vision loss were rare [16]. Another study noted that in patients with thermal corneal burns, 89% achieved full corneal recovery [17].

(c) *Radiation burns* result from UV-B absorption and damage to the corneal epithelium after prolonged exposure. UV keratitis manifests as a superficial punctuate keratitis that can easily be identified on fluorescein exam. Classically, symptoms of pain, foreign body sensation, conjunctival injection, and blepharospasm arise in a delayed fashion 6–12 h after exposure to UV light. Visual acuity may be mildly decreased. The cornea rapidly re-epithelializes with supportive treatment, and symptoms generally resolve within 24–72 h [6, 18].

2. *Ocular bodily fluid exposures* are categorized as mucocutaneous exposures. Most occupational exposures to blood transpire from needle sticks; however, in one study, eye splashes made up 17% of exposures in emergency medicine residents [19]. The typical infectious agents of concern are HIV, HBV, and HCV. Blood, serum, plasma, semen, vaginal, amniotic, pleural, peritoneal, pericardial, synovial, and cerebrospinal fluids are all capable of transmitting HIV, HBV, and HCV. Saliva is known to transmit HBV and HCV, but HIV only if the saliva contains blood. For each of these, the estimated risk of disease transmission via mucocutaneous route is relatively low, especially compared to percutaneous exposures. The estimated risk of HIV after mucous membrane exposures is 0.09% [11]. The exact risk of HBV and HCV after eye splash is not known, although there have been case reports of transmission [20, 21].

3. *Cyanoacrylate/super glue* has the ability to bond a number of materials in a matter of seconds. Super glue itself is not

known to be toxic to the eye; in fact, Dermabond®, a common cyanoacrylate, is often used in ophthalmic surgeries. Exposure generally results in false tarsorrhaphy (adherence of the upper and lower eyelids) and occasionally adheres to the cornea, which may result in a corneal abrasion if hardened glue particles scrape the cornea with blinking or eye movement [9, 22]. Ocular super glue exposures have an excellent prognosis.

Management

The common pathway for eye burns and exposures is irrigation with generous amounts of fluid. Considerations for specific injuries are noted below.

Chemical Burns

Important caveats

- *The single most important intervention for chemical exposure is prompt and copious irrigation.* Delays of even 20 s may result in permanent damage [23]. The primary goals of irrigation are normalization of pH and removal and dilution of the offending agent. Clean tap water should be used if the exposure occurs in the industrial work place, school, or home. In the ED setting, tap water should generally be avoided, as it is not sterile and contains organisms known to result in difficult-to-treat corneal ulcers. After a chemical injury, the corneal epithelium is usually absent, either partially or completely, which greatly increases the risk of infection/ulcer. Normal saline is the mainstay of treatment in the ED. Recent studies suggest that isotonic saline may not be as effective at lowering pH as newer buffering solutions. Buffering solutions such as Cederroth Eye Wash Solution, Previn, and Diphoterine are preferred and highly effective if available [24, 25]. Lactated Ringer's solution and balanced salt solutions (BSS) are also options.

- Irrigation should occur with the eyelids retracted. This can be accomplished with the assistance of an eyelid speculum or Morgan Lens. There are no specific guidelines for the amount and duration of irrigation. The amount and duration will depend on the chemical involved. Amounts up to 20 L may be necessary [26]. A common practice is to irrigate for 30 min and then stop to evaluate ocular pH level. pH should be evaluated by touching litmus paper to the fornix 5 min after discontinuing irrigation. A full ophthalmologic evaluation should occur once pH remains within the physiologic range for 30 min after irrigation cessation [27].
- Topical anesthesia with 0.5% proparacaine may allow for easier irrigation [6, 27]. Systemic analgesics may be considered.
- Apply a topical antibiotic ointment, such as erythromycin.
- Preservative-free artificial tears should be used generously.
- Topical corticosteroids, cycloplegics, doxycycline, and ascorbic acid may be used with consultation with an ophthalmologist.
- Lime and cement dust materials comprised of calcium oxide react with water to produce calcium hydroxide, which has a pH of 12.4 and can continue to cause damage. Care should be taken to remove all particles before full irrigation [14].

Hydrofluoric acid treatment is complicated by the possibility that saline and water do not control the corrosive nature of HF. One percent calcium gluconate may be a better solution as it binds the F^- ions. Calcium chloride should not be used as it has been shown to cause corneal abrasions. Hexafluorine is a novel solution engineered specifically for the treatment of HF and is beneficial if available [15].

Thermal Burns

- As in chemical burns, treatment of ocular thermal burns begins with copious irrigation. This serves to cool the eye and remove debris.
- Generous use of artificial tears and antibiotic ointment is paramount, especially if eyelid contractures result in lagophthalmos and corneal exposure [16, 28].

Radiation

- Treatment is mainly supportive. Mild oral analgesics and artificial tears are the mainstay. Artificial tears with antioxidative properties such as Artelac EDO® are recommended [18].
- Topical antibiotics (erythromycin 0.5%) are recommended.
- Topical anesthetics may be used in the setting of the exam but should not be prescribed for prolonged use without consultation.
- Cycloplegic drops and patching are not recommended [6, 18].

Bodily Fluid Exposure

- Immediately irrigate eyes with clean water, saline, or sterile irrigation solutions.
- Report the exposure to the occupational health or infectious disease departments, who can help direct postexposure treatment.
- HBV—vaccination and documented hepatitis B immune globulin are effective in preventing disease in the exposed patient.
- HCV—there is no HCV vaccination or postexposure treatment available.
- HIV—postexposure prophylaxis (PEP) should be initiated without delay when a possible exposure has

occurred. PEP is not likely to be effective after 72 h. The CDC currently recommends a regimen of three antiretroviral medications. The exact regimen should be directed by established hospital protocols and likely with expert infectious disease consultation. However, the current preferred PEP regimen consists of:

- Raltegravir 400 mg PO twice daily plus Truvada (tenofovir 300 mg + emtricitabine 200 mg) PO once daily [29].

Cyanoacrylates

- If possible, retract the eyelids and irrigate immediately. This may not be possible due to the fast-acting nature of super glue.
- Specifically for Dermabond®, the product package insert notes that polymerization of the adhesive may be accelerated by water. Wiping excess glue with dry sterile gauze followed by irrigation may be beneficial.
- For tarsorrhaphy, saturate sterile eye pads with warm tap water and apply a tight pressure patch to the eye, treat pain as necessary, and observe. Other fluids such as 3% sodium bicarbonate and mineral oil have also been used successfully. Lids will separate in 12–72 h. Cutting eyelashes is not recommended [9, 10, 22].
- For a partial tarsorrhaphy, a petroleum jelly-soaked cotton swab can be placed gently in the interpalpebral fissure and slowly slid horizontally along the inner eyelash border to aid in separating the eyelids [9].
- For damage to the cornea, treat per corneal abrasion protocol (see Chap. 7 of this book).

Disposition

- All but the most minor chemical and thermal burns require immediate consultation with an ophthalmologist.

- Bodily fluid exposures will follow up with infectious disease or occupational health as per hospital protocol.
- Patients with minor radiation burns and cyanoacrylate exposures should follow up with an ophthalmologist in 24–48 h.

Pearls/Pitfalls

- Check online sources, such as https://pubchem.ncbi.nlm.nih.gov, for Material Safety Data Sheets (MSDS) that contain detailed information on chemical properties.
- Poison control may be contacted to identify components of common household products and other chemical solutions.
- Many companies can be directly contacted and have a safety officer available who can offer product-specific advice.
- Irrigation can be aided with commercial products (Morgan Lens), or an irrigation system can be created using materials commonly found in the ED. A nasal cannula directed into the corners of the eyes may be used. The nasal cannula can be connected to IV tubing using a mixing cannula.
- A hands-free irrigation system can be created by modifying a generic dual-lumen cannula adapter and taping the apparatus to the forehead of the patient [30].

References

1. Haring RS, Sheffield ID, Channa R, Canner JK, Schneider EB. Epidemiologic trends of chemical ocular burns in the United States. JAMA Ophthalmol. 2016;134(10):1119–24.
2. Schrage N, Burgher F, Blomet J, Bodson L, Gerard M, Hall A, Josset P, Mathieu L, Merle H. Chemical ocular burns: new understanding and treatments. Berlin: Springer; 2011.

3. Lollgen RM, Lu VH, Middlebrook L, Gunja N, McCaskill M. Party bubbles: friend or foe? A conjunctival burn in a paediatric emergency department. Emerg Med Australas. 2014;26:314–5.

4. Ratnapalan S, Das L. Causes of eye burns in children. Pediatr Emerg Care. 2011;27:151–6.

5. Morgan SJ. Chemical burns of the eye: causes and management. Br J Ophthalmol. 1987;71:854–7.

6. Spector J, Fernandez WG. Chemical, thermal, and biological ocular exposures. Emerg Med Clin North Am. 2008;26:125–36, vii.

7. Barnes SS, Wong W Jr, Affeldt JC. A case of severe airbag related ocular alkali injury. Hawaii J Med Public Health. 2012;71:229–31.

8. Desai SP, Teggihalli BC, Bhola R. Superglue mistaken for eye drops. Arch Dis Child. 2005;90:1193.

9. Rouvelas H, Saffra N, Rosen M. Inadvertent tarsorrhaphy secondary to Dermabond. Pediatr Emerg Care. 2000;16:346.

10. Terman SM. Treatment of ocular super glue instillation. J Trauma. 2009;66:E70–1.

11. Moran GJ. Emergency department management of blood and body fluid exposures. Ann Emerg Med. 2000;35:47–62.

12. Dua HS, King AJ, Joseph A. A new classification of ocular surface burns. Br J Ophthalmol. 2001;85:1379–83.

13. Roper-Hall MJ. Thermal and chemical burns. Trans Ophthalmol Soc U K. 1965;85:631–53.

14. Kuckelkorn R, Schrage N, Keller G, Redbrake C. Emergency treatment of chemical and thermal eye burns. Acta Ophthalmol Scand. 2002;80:4–10.

15. Atley K, Ridyard E. Treatment of hydrofluoric acid exposure to the eye. Int J Ophthalmol. 2015;8:157–61.

16. Stern JD, Goldfarb IW, Slater H. Ophthalmological complications as a manifestation of burn injury. Burns. 1996;22:135–6.

17. Fitzgerald O'Connor E, et al. Periorbital burns – a 6 year review of management and outcome. Burns. 2015;41:616–23.

18. Willmann G. Ultraviolet keratitis: from the pathophysiological basis to prevention and clinical management. High Alt Med Biol. 2015;16:277–82.

19. Lee CH, Carter WA, Chiang WK, Williams CM, Asimos AW, Goldfrank LR. Occupational exposures to blood among emergency medicine residents. Acad Emerg Med. 1999;6:1036–43.

20. "Blood/Body Fluid Exposure Option." Blood/Body Fluid Exposure Option, 1 Jan. 2013, www.cdc.gov/nhsn/PDFs/HPS-manual/exposure/3-HPS-Exposure-options.pdf.

21. "Exposure to Blood What Healthcare Personnel Need to Know." Exposure to Blood What Healthcare Personnel Need to Know, July 2003, www.cdc.gov/HAI/pdfs/bbp/Exp_to_Blood.pdf.
22. Raynor LA. Treatment for inadvertent cyanoacrylate tarsorrhaphy: case report. Arch Ophthalmol. 1988;106:1033.
23. Rihawi S, Frentz M, Becker J, Reim M, Schrage NF. The consequences of delayed intervention when treating chemical eye burns. Graefes Arch Clin Exp Ophthalmol. 2007;245:1507–13.
24. Rihawi S, Frentz M, Reim M, Schrage NF. Rinsing with isotonic saline solution for eye burns should be avoided. Burns. 2008;34:1027–32.
25. Rihawi S, Frentz M, Schrage NF. Emergency treatment of eye burns: which rinsing solution should we choose? Graefes Arch Clin Exp Ophthalmol. 2006;244:845–54.
26. Fish R, Davidson RS. Management of ocular thermal and chemical injuries, including amniotic membrane therapy. Curr Opin Ophthalmol. 2010;21:317–21.
27. Pokhrel PK, Loftus SA. Ocular emergencies. Am Fam Physician. 2007;76:829–36.
28. Constable JD, Carroll JM. The emergency treatment of the exposed cornea in thermal burns. Plast Reconstr Surg. 1970;46: 309–12.
29. Kuhar DT, et al. Updated US Public Health Service guidelines for the management of occupational exposures to human immunodeficiency virus and recommendations for postexposure prophylaxis. Infect Control Hosp Epidemiol. 2013;34:875–92.
30. Wade RG, Peacock D. Bilateral eye irrigation: a simple and effective hands-free technique. Eur J Emerg Med. 2014;21:305–7.

Chapter 13
Ophthalmologic Procedures

Walter Green

Foreign Body Removal

Brief Introduction

Ocular foreign bodies may present on the conjunctiva, under the lids, on the cornea, or as an object that has penetrated the globe. Once identified, any globe penetration or intraocular foreign body should result in an immediate ophthalmology consultation. This discussion will focus on non-penetrating foreign bodies.

The patient's history may reveal concerns about ocular foreign bodies. Common causes of serious eye injury include work-related trauma, hammering on metal, cutting grass, grinding, sawdust, traffic accidents, and fireworks [1, 2]. Other, more rare injuries, include thorns and insect stings with retained stingers.

Whenever the equipment is available, the proper examination of the eye in the emergency department requires the use of a slit lamp. Foreign body penetration of the globe can lack

W. Green, MD
Department of Emergency Medicine, University of Texas
Southwestern Medical School, Dallas, TX, USA

© Springer International Publishing AG, part of Springer Nature 2018
B. Long, A. Koyfman (eds.), *Handbook of Emergency Ophthalmology*, https://doi.org/10.1007/978-3-319-78945-3_13

obvious clinical signs, and the diagnosis may be quite difficult [3, 4]. Transparent foreign bodies are difficult to visualize and may only be noted on careful slit-lamp examination [5].

Indications

A thorough eye examination that discovers a foreign body requires the prompt removal of the entity to preserve vision and promote rapid healing with minimal complications. The discovery of globe penetration necessitates emergent ophthalmologic consultation. Foreign bodies that do not penetrate the globe should be removed by the emergency physician. Rarely do they require the involvement of a specialist in the ED.

Equipment

Topical anesthetic—ophthalmic tetracaine or proparacaine.
    Cotton tipped swabs.
    Eye spud or sterile 25 gauge needle.
    Needle driver or 21 gauge needle.
    Slit lamp.
    Corneal burr (Algerbrush™).

Procedure

Upper Lid Foreign Body

The upper lid should be everted to search for a foreign body adhered to the conjunctiva. With the patient supine, the examiner should gently place a cotton tipped swab on the upper lid. Grasping the upper lid by the lashes, the lid can be carefully pulled away from the globe, and with the swab at the superior aspect of the tarsal plate, the upper lid is everted over the swab. The patient can aid in the maneuver by maintaining a downward gaze (Figs. 13.1 and 13.2).

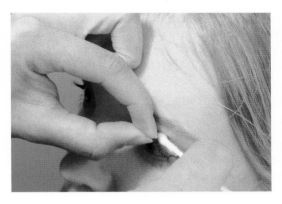

FIGURE 13.1 A cotton swab is placed on the upper lid while the examiner grasps the uppers lashes

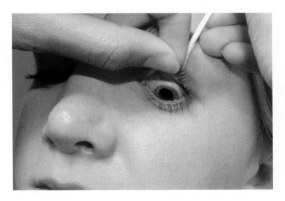

FIGURE 13.2 The upper lid is everted and the patient maintains a downward gaze

A bright light source will aid in identification and location of small foreign bodies on the upper lid. Using magnifying loupes or everting the lids while the patient is in the slit lamp will also help locate very small objects. When the foreign body is identified on the upper lid, it can typically be removed with a second clean swab using a gentle swiping motion. The upper fornix should also be gently swept, while the lid is everted, with a moistened swab and examined for any foreign body. The lower lid does not require eversion for adequate visualization, though it should be swept with a moistened swab to remove any foreign body that may not be easily seen.

Corneal Foreign Body

Removal of a corneal foreign body should be performed with the patient positioned in a slit lamp, if at all possible. Make sure the eye is well anesthetized and apply topical anesthetic liberally. Any patient movement can result in iatrogenic injury, but when the patient is positioned in the slit lamp, the risk of injury is reduced. When positioned in the slit lamp, most patient movement will be away from the provider's instrument that is used to remove any object on the cornea.

Many corneal and conjunctival foreign bodies can be removed by a gentle swipe with a moistened cotton tipped swab. If, after a few attempts, the object appears adhered to the cornea, more aggressive intervention is indicated. Care must be taken to resist damaging the corneal epithelium with repeated or aggressive swiping of the adhered foreign body.

If available, an eye spud may be used to remove a foreign body from the cornea. The vast majority of emergency departments do not have an eye spud available. A simple alternative can be made by the emergency physician using a 25 gauge needle and a needle driver to bend the tip 90° [6]. An alternative method involves bending the 25 gauge needle tip by inserting it into the orifice of a 21 gauge needle and forming the tip into a right angle [7]. Both methods provide the emergency physician with an instrument that will allow gentle extraction of an embedded foreign body on the corneal surface. Once the 25 gauge needle tip is bent to a 90° angle, it should be place on a 3 cc syringe for better dexterity (Figs. 13.3, 13.4, and 13.5).

A corneal foreign body that is embedded should be removed with the patient positioned in the slit lamp. The physician should rest his dominant hand, holding the 25 gauge needle with the bent tip, against the patient's maxillary prominence

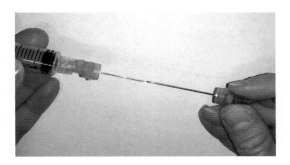

FIGURE 13.3 Inserting the tip of a 25 gauge needle into a 21 gauge needle

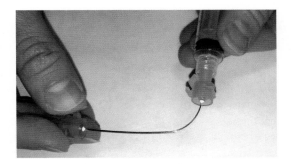

FIGURE 13.4 Bending the tip of the 25 gauge needle

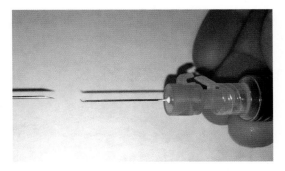

FIGURE 13.5 The finished product, a 25 gauge needle with a bent tip

or the slit-lamp forehead rest. The tip of the 25 gauge needle is carefully brought into the field of vision on the slit lamp. Once in the field of vision, the physician should advance the needle tip to the corneal foreign body, elevate the object, and remove it with the needle or with a moistened swab.

Once the foreign body is removed from the corneal, no patching is required [8]. Reexamine the patient with the slit lamp to assure that all the foreign material is removed and that none remains.

Corneal Rust Ring

Ferrous containing foreign bodies may leave behind a deposition of oxidized iron in the cornea, commonly referred to as a rust ring. Inadequate removal of a corneal rust ring is a factor in delayed healing [9]. After removal of a foreign body, slit-lamp reexamination may reveal a rust ring in the corneal cells.

With the patient still in the slit lamp and with adequate topical anesthetics, the physician can attempt to remove the remaining rust ring with an eye spud or a bent-tip 25 gauge needle. Removal will require several picking and swiping motions which can cause a large corneal defect. A preferred method is to use a commercially available corneal burr. The most commonly available instrument is the Algerbrush II™ and can be ordered over the internet for around $70 (Fig. 13.6).

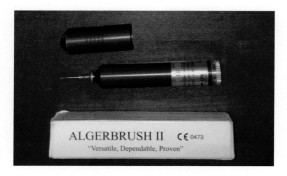

FIGURE 13.6 A corneal burr with a 1 mm disposable tip for rust ring removal

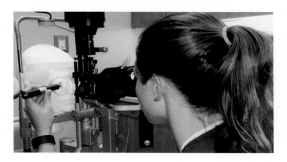

FIGURE 13.7 Use of the corneal burr with a mannequin and a chicken egg for globe simulation. Note that the physician's hand is resting on the slit-lamp chin rest for stability

The tip is disposable and has either a 1 or 0.5 mm burr. It has a small motor powered by an AA battery that stops rotating with excessive pressure. Attempts to fully remove the rust ring on the first day of presentation may be unsuccessful, and the patient should return in 24–48 h for repeat treatment with the corneal burr.

For physicians not familiar with the use of a corneal burr, several simulation models exist for training and practice. The use of a mannequin head with either gelatin or a chicken egg simulating the orbit is described in the literature and has been received with overall positive endorsements by trainees [10, 11] (Fig. 13.7).

Pearls/Pitfalls

Pearls

Slit-lamp examination is required to fully examine the globe for retained foreign body or penetration.

Foreign bodies that do not penetrate the globe should be removed by the emergency physician.

A 25 gauge needle tip can be bent to use as a foreign body removal instrument.

Rust ring removal is best accomplished with a corneal burr.

Pitfalls

Foregoing a slit-lamp examination may result in a missed foreign body or globe penetration.

Attempting to remove a corneal foreign body without positioning the patient in the slit lamp may result in corneal injury.

Patching is not required after foreign body removal.

Disposition

The use of topical antibiotics is debated and quite variable with no evidence-based studies to support or refute their use [12]. However, simple foreign bodies are still often treated with topical antibiotics as the standard of care, but ophthalmologic follow-up may not be required as most heal without difficulty [13].

As noted above, an eye patch, or a bandage contact lens, does not speed or improve healing and does not reduce pain [8]. Once very common after corneal abrasion and non-penetrating corneal foreign body removal, patching is no longer performed.

Corneal injuries are quite painful and a short course of oral narcotics are often prescribed. Topical nonsteroidal anti-inflammatory medication, specifically ketorolac ophthalmic topical drops, may also be helpful in pain control and should not delay healing in simple superficial corneal injuries [14]. All patients should be instructed to return immediately to the emergency department for increased pain, purulent discharge, worsening vision, or if not improved in 24 h. Ophthalmologic referral is appropriate for any complicated or concerning corneal foreign body.

Eye Irrigation

Brief Introduction

Chemical burns to the eye are medical emergencies and represent around 7–10% of all ocular trauma [15]. The majority of these chemical burns are occupational injuries and are a common work-related injury treated in the United States [16]. Most chemical burns to the eye are unilateral, though bilateral involvement is present in about 27% of cases [17]. Upon initial evaluation of the eye for a chemical burn and the necessary immediate irrigation, it is best to consider that both eyes have been exposed and the provider should begin bilateral irrigation. Many aspects of eye irrigation are debated and there is little evidence-based research to support specific recommendations, but immediate irrigation after exposure is one of the few common areas of agreement [18, 19]. The speed and rapidity of instituting initial eye irrigation has the greatest influence on the outcome of chemical and thermal burns to the eye [20].

The two main classes of chemicals that damage the globe are acids and alkalis. Acids cause less severe injury with damage often at the surface, especially with weaker acids. Deeper layers are protected due to the coagulation of surface proteins which can prevent penetration. Stronger acids, with pH of 2.5 or less, can cause deep burns. Alkali burns are worse due to liquefactive necrosis of the surface epithelium and deeper penetration into the corneal stroma and endothelium. Alkali burns may penetrate deep enough to damage structures in the anterior segment [16].

First responders, as well as workers who use acids and alkalis in their workplace, should be aware to immediately begin irrigation with any clean solution. Tap water is usually the most readily available and, even though hypotonic, has obvious benefits when used quickly [20].

The exposed eye(s) should be immediately placed under a stream of tap water (or irrigation solution) at the scene, and the lids should be held open to assist dilution and removal of the offending agent.

Commercial solutions, normal saline (NS), and lactated Ringer's (LR) have all been employed with success though there are no good evidence-based studies to determine which is best. Normal saline has a pH of about 6.5, while lactated Ringer's has a pH closer to 7.0, though actual pH can vary with different lot numbers and production times [21, 22]. Most sources prefer to recommend LR for the most comfortable irrigating solution—and warm LR is considered even better if immediately available [23].

Irrigation by first responders or in the emergency department can be achieved by several methods. Until the 1970s, irrigation was performed by directing a stream of irrigation fluid into the eye by one provider, while the second held the lids open manually, with lid retractors or with eye specula. Around 1970, Dr. Morgan developed the Morgan Therapeutic Lens while treating patients during the Vietnam War, and it became available in the United States for use, though each lens currently costs around $35 ($70 for bilateral irrigation) [24]. The Morgan Lens allows irrigation of the eye through a plastic contact lens that connects to a standard IV set. A simpler method, using a $0.50 nasal cannula taped at the bridge of the nose, can allow delivery of irrigation fluid to both eyes at the medial canthi. There are no randomized studies to indicate which method is the best or most effective.

There is no consensus regarding either duration of irrigation or the appropriate amount of irrigation solution that should be used [18]. Most ophthalmologists agree that irrigation should be performed for 30 min and the pH of the tears in the inferior fornix should be tested. If the pH is not close to 7.4, another 30 min of irrigation should follow. The process should continue with testing every 30 min until pH returns to normal [16].

Indications

Any concern over significant foreign body contamination to the eye should alert the emergency physician to consider immediate irrigation. Not all irritants and harmful chemical exposures will present with a clear history and an obvious declaration that the globe or its contents are at risk for injury. For example, older automobile airbags powered by the propellant sodium azide produced sodium hydroxide with a resultant potential devastating alkali exposure. Similarly, sparklers contain magnesium hydroxide, and direct eye exposure can cause severe damage and vision loss [16]. Therefore, any suspicion of alkali or acid exposure is an indication for irrigation for 30 min with subsequent pH testing.

The CDC recommends irrigation of the eye for biologic exposures, especially if exposed to blood to reduce transmission of infectious agents including hepatitis and HIV. The CDC lists irrigation fluid as clean water, saline, or sterile irrigants, though there is no specific suggestion about methodology, amount of irrigant, or duration of irrigation [25].

Equipment

Clean irrigation solution—warm lactated Ringer's in IV bags, if available.
   Cotton tipped swabs.
   Topical anesthetic: tetracaine or proparacaine.
   IV tubing, connectors, and tape.
   pH paper.
   Towels and a wastebasket to collect irrigation fluid.
   Morgan Therapeutic Lens—OR.
   Standard nasal oxygen cannula with 4 × 4 gauze and scissors.

Procedure

First responders and emergency department personnel should be trained to immediately begin irrigation of the eyes for any chemical exposure. The patient should be placed supine with the head down, if possible, and immediate flush of the eyes should proceed with the first available clean solution. Tap water is the obvious, readily available irrigant in most situations.

Emergency department treatment should begin with a topical anesthetic, using either topical tetracaine or proparacaine, to easy comfort and to reduce blepharospasm so that irrigation can be performed with greater success. If topical anesthetics are not immediately available, irrigation should proceed while the medication is retrieved.

At first inspection, if any gross foreign bodies or chemical contaminants are noted, they should quickly and gently be removed with moistened cotton tipped swabs. The upper lids should quickly be everted and swept with a moistened swab, followed by retraction of the lower lid which should also be swept.

Irrigation can be accomplished by several methods. Using two personnel, one person directs irrigation solution into the eyes while the lids are retracted and held open with lid retractors by one or two other providers. Though this is the classic description of eye irrigation, it is uncomfortable, requires at least two (or three) providers, and is generally impracticable.

The two most expedient methods for eye irrigation involve using either a standard nasal oxygen cannula for irrigant delivery or a Morgan Therapeutic Lens. To irrigate the eyes using a nasal cannula, it should be placed over the head, with each cannula resting at the bridge of the nose and directed toward the medial canthus of each eye (Fig. 13.8).

Gauze 4 × 4 s can be placed laterally to displace the tubing away from the palpebral fissures and improve comfort. If necessary, the cannula can be taped in place at the brow and laterally to maintain position, though often tape is not required. Using scissors, the connector can be cut and discarded so that standard IV tubing may be inserted into the nasal cannula for irrigation fluid (Figs. 13.9 and 13.10).

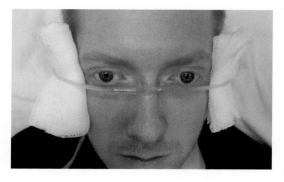

Figure 13.8 Nasal cannula in place over the bridge of the nose and 4 × 4 gauze placed laterally to move the tubing away from the palpebral fissures and eye lashes

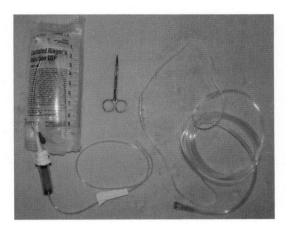

FIGURE 13.9 Lactated Ringer's, IV tubing, scissors, and a nasal cannula

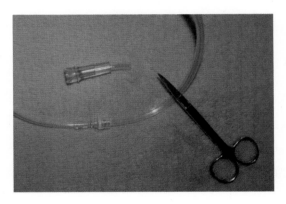

FIGURE 13.10 Nasal cannula wall connector cut off to allow for IV tubing insertion

Warm lactated Ringer's, or another available clean irrigant solution, should be hung and irrigation begun quickly with the patient in the supine, head-down position. With the head down, the irrigation solution will run off the stretcher and should be collected in a wastebasket. The patient should be encouraged to look up, down, left, and right during irrigation,

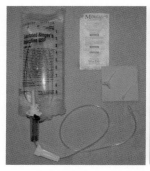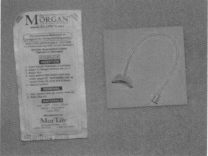

FIGURE 13.11 A Morgan Therapeutic Lens, lactated Ringer's, and IV tubing; Morgan Lens enlarged

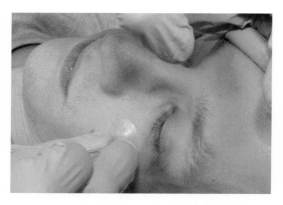

FIGURE 13.12 The patient is looking down, preparing for the Morgan Lens insertion

while the irrigant flows from the medial canthus bilaterally and cleanses each eye.

A Morgan Therapeutic Lens can be inserted in each eye for irrigation if the provider chooses this method over a nasal cannula (Fig. 13.11). Each lens should be connected to warm lactated Ringer's or other irrigation solution, and a low rate of flow started before insertion. The patient should look down while the provider grasps the upper eyelashes and lid, and the lens should be inserted under the upper lid (Figs. 13.12

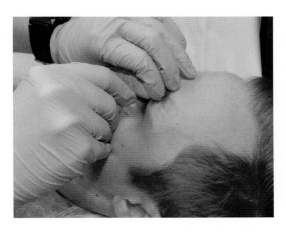

FIGURE 13.13 The upper lid is grasped for insertion of the lens under the upper lid

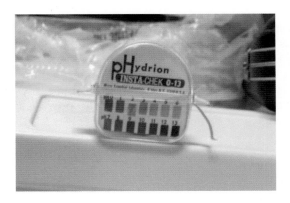

FIGURE 13.14 pH paper

and 13.13). After releasing the upper lid, the patient should look up, and the provider should retract the lower lid and drop the lens in place. The flow rate can then be increased to the desired level. Some patient prefer to have the tubing taped to their cheeks for comfort.

After 30 min of irrigation, pH paper should be used for pH testing in each eye (Fig. 13.14).

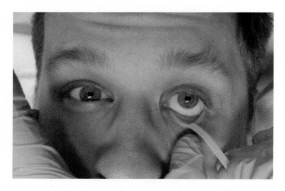

FIGURE 13.15 pH testing of the patient's tears by contacting the lower lid conjunctiva

The lower lid should be retracted and the paper should be held against the lid conjunctiva to sample the tears. If pH has not normalized, perform 30 more minutes of irrigation with pH testing again. The cycle should continue until the pH returns to normal. For severe alkali burns, 2 or 3 h of irrigation may be required. A final pH test should also be repeated 20 min after irrigation has ceased to assure that no rebound from retained chemicals occurred. If there is any concern about the accuracy of the pH paper, the providers can use their own tears as a normal control [15] (Fig. 13.15).

Pearls/Pitfalls

Pearls

Immediately irrigate the eyes for any significant concern about chemical exposure.

Begin with bilateral irrigation if there is any question about bilateral exposure.

Use the first available clean solution for irrigation, whether tap water, D5W, normal saline, or lactated Ringer's. Changing to lactated Ringer's can be done soon thereafter, but there should be no delay in initial irrigation.

Pitfalls

Delaying irrigation to "find the right solution," to warm the solution, to consult with EMS, or to get advice from a colleague should never occur.

Halting irrigation before pH returns to normal may cause severe damage to the eye.

Disposition

After adequate irrigation to return pH to normal, the eye should be thoroughly reexamined with fluorescein and a slit lamp. Any concern for significant chemical injury demands emergent consultation with ophthalmology.

Lateral Canthotomy

Brief Introduction

Orbital compartment syndrome occurs when pressure in the orbit impairs the normal perfusion of the optic nerve with resultant optic nerve ischemia and blindness [26]. The majority of cases of orbital compartment syndrome, and the emergent need for a lateral canthotomy, are secondary to trauma.

The most common cause of loss of vision in children, excluding congenital problems, is due to trauma [27]. Likewise, orbital trauma in adults ranks high as a significant cause of blindness. The emergency physician must be ready to intervene to reduce orbital compartment syndrome to preserve vision in children or adults.

The orbit is a cone-shaped structure bordered by stiff bony walls, and it contains the globe and retrobulbar tissues. Anteriorly, the eyelids and canthal tendons form a somewhat immobile boundary. The medial and lateral canthal tendons are fibrous structures that attach the eyelids to the orbital rim.

The canthal tendons function to limit any significant anterior displacement of the globe. Although small increases in orbital volume can be compensated for by forward displacement of the globe and prolapse of fat, a rapid rise in intraorbital pressure normally ensues [28].

Indications

The most common cause of increased orbital compartment pressures, with resultant retrobulbar hemorrhage and reduction of optic nerve perfusion, is trauma to the globe and the contents of the orbit. However, the emergency physician should be aware of other situations that may cause orbital compartment syndrome. Recent facial surgery including frontal sinus irrigation, endoscopic sinus surgery [29], neoplasms [30], superficial facial burns [31], excessive fluid resuscitation of major burns [32], coagulopathies (e.g., cirrhotics) with spontaneous retrobulbar bleeding [33], complications of transvenous embolization of carotid-cavernous fistulas [34], subarachnoid hemorrhage [35], spontaneous bleeding from orbital varices [36], and traumatic asphyxia [37] have all been reported as causes of orbital compartment syndrome successfully treated with lateral canthotomy.

Presenting symptoms and signs will include loss of vision in the affected eye and a dramatic decline in visual acuity associated with pain. An afferent pupillary defect, where the pupil constricts when light is directed in the opposite eye but not the affected eye (Marcus-Gunn), may be noted. Chemosis, periorbital edema, abnormal extraocular movement or ophthalmoparesis, and proptosis are also common findings [38]. Proptosis is best recognized when the examiner is in the "bird's eye position," standing at the head of the bed while the patient is supine and the examiner can look over the frontal bone onto the zygomatic arches and observe for bulging of either orbit. Emergency physicians are familiar with this position, assumed when preparing to use direct laryngoscopy for oral intubation.

Increased intraocular pressure is present in orbital compartment syndrome, but there is no literature to support using tonometry measurements alone as an indication for lateral canthotomy [39]. Generally, pressures at or above 40 mm Hg are an indication for emergent intervention [40]. Imaging is not required before canthotomy and can delay appropriate and rapid intervention. Both CT and MRI can reveal a retrobulbar hematoma and tenting of the posterior globe, but those findings are not sensitive or reliable.

Remember: indications for lateral canthotomy include vision loss, pain, proptosis, and concern for orbital compartment syndrome with resultant optic nerve ischemia. The procedure should be performed under 2 h from the time of the optic nerve insult and before imaging.

Equipment

Chlorhexidine or alcohol to cleanse the skin and lateral canthus.

Sterile saline and a large syringe for irrigation and debris removal.

1% lidocaine with 1:100,000 epinephrine, 2 ml.

Small syringe for injection equipped with a 25 gauge needle.

Hemostats, sterile.

Sharp small scissors, sterile.

Forceps, preferably toothed to reduce tissue damage, sterile.

Sterile gloves and towels for drapes.

Tonometer to check pressures, but not required.

Procedure

With the patient either supine, or if possible with the head elevated to reduce intraocular pressures, the skin at the lateral canthus is cleansed with chlorhexidine or alcohol while avoiding chemical injury to the globe and conjunctiva. Since many of these injuries are related to trauma and contaminated,

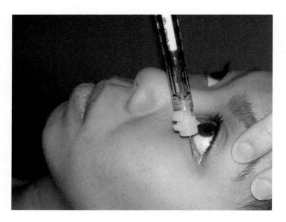

FIGURE 13.16 Injection of lidocaine with needle aimed toward the edge of the bony orbital rim

debris in the eye and under the lids may be removed with quick normal saline irrigation.

If time permits, small sterile towels should be placed to allow for a clean field. The skin at the lateral canthus is infiltrated with 1–2 ml of 1% lidocaine with 1:100,000 epinephrine. The 25 gauge needle should be directed laterally, avoiding the globe, and infiltration continued in the tissue until contact is made with the bone at the orbital rim. Local anesthesia is accomplished after a pause of 1–2 min (Fig. 13.16).

Next, the hemostat is used to crush the tissue at the lateral canthus to reduce bleeding. One arm of the hemostat is placed inside the palpebral fissure and directed posteriorly, and the other arm is placed on the skin (Fig. 13.17). Clamp the hemostat and leave it in place for 1 min, then remove it (Fig. 13.18).

Sharp small sterile scissors are used to perform the canthotomy. The tissue is cut with the incision directed posteriorly and should extend a full 1 cm toward the lateral bony orbital rim. Be careful to direct the scissors away from the globe to prevent any globe injury (Fig. 13.19).

The final steps are the most critical and therapeutic. Using a toothed forcep, the lower lid should be gently retracted to expose the inferior crus of the lateral canthal tendon. Edema and tissue distortion from trauma may make identification

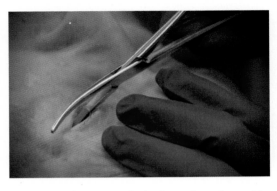

FIGURE 13.17 Preparing to crush the lateral canthus with a pair of hemostats

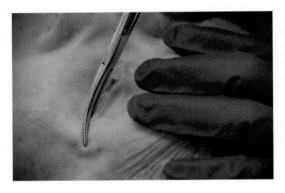

FIGURE 13.18 Clamping and crushing the tissue for 1 min with the hemostats

difficult, so gentle blunt dissection at the inferior and lateral aspect of the orbit with the scissors can help identify the tendon. The operator can feel the tendon or "strum" it with the scissors, much like the feel of a guitar string [41] (Fig. 13.20).

Using the scissors, the inferior crus of the lateral tendon is cut with a 1 cm incision, again directed laterally and inferiorly away from the globe. The lower lid should now be lax and allow the globe to displace inferiorly and laterally to reduce pressure (Fig. 13.22).

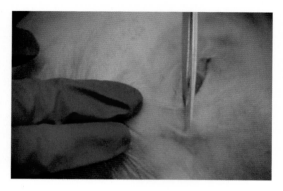

FIGURE 13.19 Preparing to incise the lateral canthus with small sharp scissors

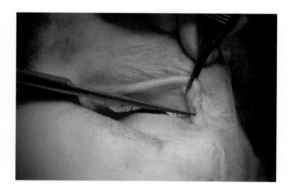

FIGURE 13.20 Lateral canthotomy completed, with the lid retracted to expose the inferior canthal ligament, so that cantholysis can be performed

Intraocular pressure should be checked if a tonometer is available. The pressure should fall below 40 mm Hg. Clinical reassessment should discover resolution of any afferent pupillary defect as optic nerve ischemia resolves. Visual acuity should also improve. If there is a concern that pressure has not been reduced, the superior crus of the lateral canthal tendon should be located and resected as well, though often resection of the inferior crus alone is adequate. If intraocular pressure continues to remain high, ophthalmologic intervention in the operating room may be required, as long as other emergent traumatic injuries will allow intercession.

Pearls/Pitfalls

Pearls

Recognize facial trauma as the leading cause of orbital compartment syndrome.

Indications for cantholysis include painful vision loss, afferent pupillary defect, proptosis, and loss of extraocular movements.

Lateral canthotomy and cantholysis should be accomplished within 2 h of optic nerve ischemia.

Pitfalls

Delaying treatment to obtain CT or MRI images should never occur.

Performing lateral canthotomy, but failing to fully divide the inferior canthal tendon, will not relieve intraocular pressure.

Globe injury due to misdirection of scissors when performing the lateral canthotomy, or lateral canthus tendon division, must be avoided.

Disposition

Ophthalmology consultation is required after lateral canthotomy for continued intraocular pressure observation, repair, and follow-up. If the lateral canthotomy was properly performed, repair should be simple and without significant complications. When appropriate, ophthalmology consultation can be obtained before the initial intervention—but there should be no delay in lateral canthotomy by the emergency physician. There is no purpose in speaking with a consultant who may be too far away to intervene rapidly.

If orbital compartment syndrome is not relieved by lateral canthotomy and division of the lateral canthal tendon, emergent operative intervention by an ophthalmologist is the

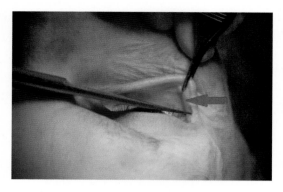

FIGURE 13.21 The arrow points toward the inferior canthal ligament. Usually it is not visible due to swelling, and it must be felt by "strumming" with the scissors

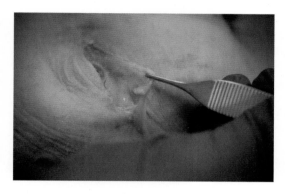

FIGURE 13.22 The lateral canthotomy and inferior cantholysis is complete with a lax lower lid

definitive next step. Unfortunately, emergent operative intervention for other traumatic injuries may take precedence with resultant vision loss in the affected eye.

The author acknowledges Natalie Sciano MD, Samantha Sales MD, John Corker MD, Ashley Phipps MD, and William Fox MD for their assistance with Figs. 13.1, 13.2, 13.3, 13.4, 13.5, 13.6, 13.7, 13.8, 13.9, 13.10, 13.11, 13.12, 13.13, 13.14, 13.15, and 13.16. Figures 13.17, 13.18, 13.19, 13.20, 13.21, and 13.22 are credited to Fernando Benitez MD.

References

1. George J, Ali N, Rahman NA, Joshi N. Spectrum of intra-ocular foreign bodies and the outcome of their management in Brunei. Int Ophthalmol. 2013;33(3):277–84.
2. Choovuthayakorn J, Hansapinyo L, Ittipunkul N, Patikulsila D, Kunavisarut P. Predictive factors and outcomes of posterior segment intraocular foreign bodies. Eye (Lond). 2011;25(12):1622–6.
3. Mostafavi D, Olumba K, Shrier EM. Fiberglass intraocular foreign body with no initial ocular symptoms. Retin Cases Brief Rep. 2014;8(1):10–2.
4. Lapira M, Karl D, Murgatroyd H. Siderosis bulbi as a consequence of a missed intraocular foreign body. BMJ Case Rep. 2014. https://doi.org/10.1136/bcr-2013-202904.
5. Bansal R, Jain AK, Sanghi G. Polyethylene foreign body on the cornea. Cornea. 2008;27(5):605–8.
6. Beyer H, Cherkas D. Corneal foreign body removal using a bent needle tip. Am J Emerg Med. 2012;30(3):489–90.
7. Lim LT, Al-Ani A, Ramaesh K. Simple innovative measures for ease of corneal foreign body removal. Ann Acad Med Singapore. 2011;40(10):469–70.
8. Menghini M, Knecht PB, Kaufmann C, Kovacs R, Watson SL, Landau K, Bosch MM. Treatment of traumatic corneal abrasions: a three-arm, prospective, randomized study. Ophthalmic Res. 2013;50(1):13–8.
9. Jayamanne DG, Bell RW. Non-penetrating corneal foreign body injuries: factors affecting delay in rehabilitation of patients. J Accid Emerg Med. 1994;11(3):195–7.
10. Austin PE, Ljung M, Dunn KA. A new model for teaching corneal foreign body removal. Acad Emerg Med. 1995;2(9):831–4.
11. Cassara M, Tenner KR, Borheck A. The incredible embeddable egg: an inexpensive model for simulating corneal foreign bodies and teaching slit lamp-associated skills. Acad Emerg Med. 2011;18(5 Suppl. 1):S255.
12. Sharma M, McLeod SL, Shah A. The use of antibiotics in corneal abrasion and corneal foreign bodies in the emergency department. Can J Emerg Med. 2013;15:S4.
13. Brissette A, Mednick Z, Baxter S. Evaluating need for close follow-up after removal of a noncomplicated corneal foreign body. Cornea. 2014;33(11):1193–6.
14. Weaver CS, Terrell KM. Evidence-based emergency medicine. Update: do ophthalmic nonsteroidal anti-inflammatory drugs

reduce the pain associated with simple corneal abrasion without delaying healing? Ann Emerg Med. 2003;41(1):134–40.

15. Connor AJ, Severn P. Use of a control to aid pH assessment of chemical eye injuries. Emerg Med J. 2009;26(11):811–2.

16. Spector J, Fernandez WG. Chemical, thermal, and biological ocular exposures. Emerg Med Clin North Am. 2008;26(1):125–36.

17. Wade RG, Peacock D. Bilateral eye irrigation: a simple and effective hands-free technique. Eur J Emerg Med. 2014;21(4):305–7.

18. Chau JP, Lee DT, Lo SH. A systematic review of methods of eye irrigation for adults and children with ocular chemical burns. Worldviews Evid Based Nurs. 2012;9(3):129–38.

19. Kuckelkorn R, Schrage N, Keller G, Redbrake C. Emergency treatment of chemical and thermal eye burns. Acta Ophthalmol Scand. 2002;80(1):4–10.

20. Ikeda N, Hayasaka S, Hayasaka Y, Wantanabe K. Alkali burns of the eye: effect of immediate copious irrigation with tap water on their severity. Ophthalmologica. 2006;220(4):225–8.

21. Jones JB, Schoenleber DB, Gillen JP. The tolerability of lactated Ringer's solution and BSS plus for ocular irrigation with and without the Morgan therapeutic lens. Acad Emerg Med. 1998;5(12):1150–6.

22. Saidinejad M, Burns MM. Ocular alternatives in pediatric emergency medicine. Pediatr Emerg Care. 2005;21(1):23–6.

23. Duffy B. Managing chemical eye injuries. Emerg Nurse. 2008;16(1):25–9.

24. Bixby S. Dr. Morgan Bio. The morgan lens. MorTan, Inc. http://morganlens.com/?s=Dr.+Morgan. Accessed 7 Oct 2016.

25. Centers for Disease Control and Prevention. Exposure to blood. 2003. http://www.cdc.gov/hai/pdfs/bbp/exp_to_blood.pdf. Accessed 7 Oct 2016.

26. Mohammadi F, Rashan A, Psaltis A, Janisewicz A, Li P, El-Sawy T, Nayak JV. Intraocular pressure changes in emergent surgical decompression of orbital compartment syndrome. JAMA Otolaryngol Head Neck Surg. 2015;141(6):562–5.

27. Messman AM. Ocular injuries: new strategies in emergency department management. Emerg Med Pract. 2015;17(11):1–21.

28. Carrim ZI, Anderson IW, Kyle PM. Traumatic orbital compartment syndrome: importance of prompt recognition and management. Eur J Emerg Med. 2007;14(3):174–6.

29. Colletti G, Fogagnolo P, Alleyi F, Rabbiosi D, Bebi V, Rossetti L, Chiapasco M, Felisati G. Retrobulbar hemorrhage during or after endonasal or periorbital surgery: what to do, when and how to do it. J Craniofac Surg. 2015;26(3):897–901.

30. See A, Gan EC. Orbital compartment syndrome during endoscopic drainage of subperiosteal orbital abscess. Am J Otolaryngol. 2015;36(6):828–31.
31. Hurst J, Johnson D, Campbell R, Baxter S, Kratky V. Orbital compartment syndrome in a burn patient without aggressive fluid resuscitation. Orbit. 2014;33(5):375–7.
32. Sullivan SR, Ahmadi AJ, Singh CN, Sires BS, Engray LH, Gibran NS, Heinbach DM, Klein MB. Elevated orbital pressure: another untoward effect of massive resuscitation after burn injury. J Trauma. 2006;60(1):72–6.
33. Nemiroff J, Baharestani S, Juthani VV, Klein KS, Zoumalan C. Cirrhosis-related coagulopathy resulting in disseminated intravascular coagulation and spontaneous orbital hemorrhages. Orbit. 2014;33(5):372–4.
34. Sia PI, Sia DIT, Scroop R, Selva D. Orbital compartment syndrome following transvenous embolization of carotid-cavernous fistula. Orbit. 2014;33(1):52–4.
35. Colak S, Erdogan MO, Duran L, Kati C, Senel A. Retrobulbar hemorrhage associated with subarachnoid hemorrhage. J Exp Clin Med. 2013;30(4):373–5.
36. Haizul IM, Kiet-Phang L, Kalthum UMN. Reversal of blindness in haemorrhagic orbital varices by prompt orbital decompression. J Neurooncol. 2012;36:45–6.
37. Prodhan P, Noviski NN, Butler WE, Eskandar E, Ellen Grant P, Whalen MJ. Orbital compartment syndrome mimicking cerebral herniation in a 12-year-old boy with severe traumatic asphyxia. Pediatr Crit Care Med. 2003;4(3):367–9.
38. Sun MT, Chan WO, Selva D. Traumatic orbital compartment syndrome: importance of the lateral canthotomy and cantholysis. Emerg Med Australas. 2014;26(3):274–8.
39. Lima V, Burt B, Leibovitch I, Prabhakaran V, Goldberg RA, Selva D. Orbital compartment syndrome: the ophthalmic surgical emergency. Surv Ophthalmol. 2009;54(4):441–9.
40. Rowh AD, Ufberg JW, Chan TC, Vilke GM, Harrigan RA. Lateral canthotomy and cantholysis: emergency management of orbital compartment syndrome. J Emerg Med. 2015;48(3):325–30.
41. Iserson KV, Luke-Blyden Z, Clemans S. Orbital compartment syndrome: alternative tools to perform a lateral canthotomy and cantholysis. Wilderness Environ Med. 2016;27(1):85–91.

Chapter 14
Ocular Ultrasound

Brian Patrick Murray

Brief Introduction

Approximately 2% of all patients present to an emergency department (ED) with an ocular complaint [1]. These complaints include self-limited benign pathologies such as conjunctivitis and severe eyesight comprising issues such as globe rupture. Ocular complaints can be stress provoking to emergency physicians in part due to the fact that eye injuries are the leading cause of monocular blindness in the United States [2–4]. Additionally, a full ocular evaluation is frequently limited by technical skill, familiarity with the examination, and specialized equipment. In fact, the non-dilated funduscopic exam is the examination skill that practitioners feel the least confident in their ability to perform [5].

Computed tomography (CT) and magnetic resonance imaging (MRI) are both able to evaluate for ocular pathology but have limitations related to radiation, duration of study, magnetic foreign bodies, and time to interpretation, and they may require the patient to leave the ED. US is portable and inexpensive and is readily used for a wide variety of situations [6–8].

B. P. Murray, DO
Emergency Medicine, Brooke Army Medical Center,
San Antonio, TX, USA

© Springer International Publishing AG, part of Springer Nature 2018
B. Long, A. Koyfman (eds.), *Handbook of Emergency Ophthalmology*, https://doi.org/10.1007/978-3-319-78945-3_14

Point-of-care ultrasound is an emerging skill in emergency medicine, allowing for goal-directed ultrasound examination to answer a specific clinical question, allowing for detailed information to be gathered through anatomical, functional, and physiologic information [9]. The human eye is an ideal organ for examination with ultrasound, as it is superficial and fluid filled, allowing for a detailed clear image with a high-frequency transducer [10]. One of the largest draws of bedside ocular ultrasound is that it is safe, easy to use, time efficient, and accurate. A 2002 study in an academic ED showed that in the hands of emergency physicians, ocular US possesses diagnostic sensitivity and specificity of 100% and 97.2%, respectively, for ocular pathology [11].

Safety

Safety is always of high concern, and bedside ultrasonography should follow the principles "as low as reasonably achievable" (ALARA). US evaluation should use the lowest amount of energy for the shortest amount of time in order to obtain images at the necessary quality [12]. Harm can be caused by ultrasound either by the absorption of the ultrasonic energy causing thermal injuries or by ultrasonic waves causing cavitation [13–15]. No studies to date have shown harm from the standard use of ultrasound [16, 17]; however, the number of applications of diagnostic US is rapidly progressing, adding additional uses at a rate that far outpaces the studies evaluating safety. The principles of ALARA should always be applied to all diagnostic scans, and only orbital-rated equipment should be used to answer the clinical question [18].

Normal Anatomy

The ocular globe is a fluid-filled sphere, which is an ideal acoustic window for US evaluation. The human eye has an antero-posterior depth of 24–25 mm, highly consistent from person to person [19]. The most superficial structure visible on US is the cornea, which presents as a thin hyperechoic arch contiguous with the sclera. Deep to the cornea is an anechoic structure representing the anterior chamber filled with aqueous humor. The anterior chamber and corresponding superficial structures (conjunctiva, sclera, cornea, iris, and ciliary bodies) of the eye are poorly resolved and difficult to evaluate with standard point-of-care US equipment; however, these structures rarely need to be emergently evaluated but can be visualized by an ophthalmologist with ultrahigh frequency ultrasound [10]. The posterior wall of the anterior chamber is composed of the hyperechoic iris and convex echo of the anterior portion of the lens. The lens is a hyperechoic outline of a biconcave structure with an anechoic center. The distal portion of the lens and the underside of the iris delineate the anterior edge of the posterior chamber, also anechoic, which is filled with viscous vitreous humor. As people age, small low-intensity reflections may be observed within the posterior chamber, which represent vitreous bodies caused by vitreous syneresis or liquefaction of the vitreous gel. At the posterior portion of the posterior chamber is the hyperechoic retina, choroid, and sclera. In the absence of pathology, it will be impossible to distinguish these layers using standard point-of-care US equipment. Deep to the retina is the posterior eye socket including the optic nerve and surrounding retro-orbital fat, which is echogenic. The echogenic optic nerve is a linear structure extending posteriorly and perpendicularly from the retina. The optic nerve itself is hypoechoic to the surrounding optic nerve sheath, which is hyperechoic. The optic nerve can be viewed longitudinally in the center of the screen with some minor adjustments of the transducer angle. The central retinal artery and vein course through the center of the optic nerve and can be identified using color flow Doppler over the distal optic nerve.

Technique

Patients should be positioned supine for an ocular US exam, but the head of the bed can be elevated if the patient is unable to tolerate the supine position. With the eyes closed, but not clenched, a copious amount of clean water-soluble ultrasound gel is applied to create a stand-off from the eye. This allows the beam to focus on the superficial anterior chamber and alleviates pressure placed on the globe. Sterile ultrasound gel can also be used and is less irritating to some individuals. The use of a thin plastic film, such as a Tegaderm™, placed over the closed eye prior to the application of the ultrasound gel can improve comfort and help prevent contamination of the conjunctiva [20]. Be aware that any air trapped under the film may degrade image quality.

The US transducer should be held in a pincer grasp by the thumb and index finger, while the other fingers and hypothenar eminence stabilize the hand by resting on the patient's maxilla, supraorbital ridge, glabella, or other bony prominence. A linear high-frequency ultrasound probe, 7–15 MHz, should be used, which provides high-resolution images. A probe with a smaller footprint will also help obtain the highest quality images, as it will fit better within the ocular bony architecture and avoid shadowing and artifacts caused by the bones surrounding the eye. B-mode is used for bedside ocular ultrasonic evaluation, as this will provide a detailed two-dimensional image of the eye. The depth should be set so that the entire posterior chamber is seen with the inclusion of 1–2 cm of the optic nerve. The gain is adjusted to ensure the posterior chamber is hypoechoic, almost to the point of being anechoic, to allow for visualization of faint echoes [21]. However, if the gain is too low, subtle pathology may be missed. If the US machine allows selection of the examination type, the use of the "ophthalmologic" or "ocular" setting will provide the best possible images while minimizing risk to the patient due to energy absorption. However, not every machine will have this setting, and in its absence, the "small parts" setting will provide similar image quality.

The standard position of the sonographer, as with all diagnostic US surveys, is to stand to the patient's right side and to hold the probe in the right hand. The eye should be evaluated in at least two separate planes, longitudinal and transverse. For examination of the longitudinal plane, the probe should be held vertically, with the probe marker cephalad. For the transverse plan, the probe should be turned 90° from the longitudinal position with the probe marker positioned to the patient's right [22]. In each plane, the probe should be fanned or moved through the entire eye to visualize the complete globe. A real-time scan through the globe should be saved, and if not available, the best 2D image identified can be saved or printed. Additionally, an image of the mid-eye plane which contains the cornea, iris, lens, vitreous body, retina, and ideally the optic nerve should be obtained. This procedure should be repeated in the opposite eye, which even in the absence of symptoms or pathology can serve as a normal comparison.

Indications/Pathology

Retinal Detachment/Vitreous Detachment

A retinal detachment (RD) occurs when there is a separation of the neurosensory retina from the underlying pigmented layer due to vitreous fluid penetration through a hole in the retinal which expands a potential space behind the retinal epithelium. Prompt recognition of this disorder is needed to save any or all of the patient's vision. Patients will typically present with the complaint of painless monocular loss or vision impairment. If there is accompanying vitreous hemorrhage, they might also describe that their visual field is obscured by "black rain." Initially a RD may be asymptomatic but will eventually progress to loss of visual acuity, or it may be described by patients as a dark shadow covering their sight [10].

A posterior vitreous detachment (PVD) is a process of lifelong vitreous liquefaction that occurs in less than 10% of patients younger than 60 years of age, 27% in patients in their seventh decade of life, and 63% of people in their 80s. Patients will complain of floaters, and 22–44% will describe "flashers" but will not typically complain of decreased vision

[23]. PVDs are a risk factor for the development of a RD but do not hold the same emergent disposition or risk of vision loss as does a RD.

Funduscopic evaluation of the retina is difficult in the emergency department setting in even the best of situations, and impossible in the worst, including inability to visualize the posterior segment due to a hyphema, cataract, or vitreous hemorrhage [24]. US has been shown to be an effective tool to emergently diagnose retinal detachments and differentiate them from PVDs, with a sensitivity of 91–100% and a specificity of 83–96% in the hands of emergency physicians [25–28].

In a normal eye without pathology, the retina is continuous with the posterior elements of the globe and is not a visibly distinct structure on US. A RD is seen as a hyperechoic membrane that may undulate with vitreous convection or with eye movements and appears to have been lifted off the posterior wall of the globe. The space between the RD and the posterior wall will appear hypoechoic to anechoic. It is important that the entire retina is evaluated to prevent missing a small RD in the periphery of the globe. The anterior most portion of the retina attaches just posterior to the ciliary bodies, and the patient may need to gaze upward or downward to adequately rule out a RD in this peripheral portion of the retina.

The retina is firmly attached to the optic disc, and as such, any RD that extends over the optic disc will be shaped like a "V." This anchoring to the optic disc is one method of differentiating a RD from a PVD. A PVD can appear similar to RD; however, there is no anchoring at the optic disc, and the separated membrane will continue over the optic disc. A PVD will also appear thinner than an RD and will have a smoother structure.

Another means of distinguishing a RD from a PVD is through color Doppler imaging (CDI). As the retina pulls away from the pigmented payer, it takes its blood supply with it, while a PVD does not have any blood vessels within the separated layer. Using CDI or spectral pulse-wave Doppler to evaluate for blood flow within the membranes floating above the posterior globe has a sensitivity of 92.3% and a specificity of 100% for the identification of a RD. Additionally, the positive predictive value is 100%, and the negative predictive value is 93.3% [29]. However, it is possible that the RD had its blood supply severed, and therefore, regardless of the sonographic appearance, it is difficult to distinguish a PVD from an RD, and therefore identification of a membrane raised off the posterior globe should prompt an ophthalmologic consultation within 24 h, or sooner if available.

Lens Dislocation

Ectopia lentis, or lens dislocation, occurs when the crystalline lens of the eye is moved from its normal position within lens patella fossa just posterior to the iris after disruption of the zonular fibers which tether the lens to the ciliary bodies and hold it in place. The most common cause is trauma [30], but it may also occur in patients with connective tissue disorders, such as Marfan or Ehlers-Danlos syndrome, or in patients with homocystinuria, aniridia, or syphilis [31]. The most common complaint associated with lens dislocation are pain, binocular and monocular diplopia, photosensitivity, and decreased vision ranging from partial and blurry vision all the way to complete loss of vision [32]. Lens dislocations primarily are the result of high energy trauma, such as motor vehicle accidents, motorcycle accidents, and pedestrians struck by motor vehicles. Diagnosis can be made by ocular CT, MRI, and US. US has the potential to be the fastest modality, as it is readily available at bedside in many emergency departments and exposes the patient to no radiation. It has a sensitivity and specificity of 84.6% and 98.3%, respectively. It performs well when compared to ocular CT, with a Cohen's kappa coefficient of 0.83 [33].

On US, a lens dislocation can be identified when the lens is not in its usual place. It may be in the anterior chamber, free floating within the posterior chamber, or laying against the retina [34]. Lens subluxation can also occur and is more difficult to diagnose. Having the patient rotate their globe during US evaluation can help detect abnormal movements of the lens and increase the likelihood of detecting a lens subluxation [35]. If a lens dislocation is identified, the US should be stopped, as this may be the only indication of a ruptured globe, the eye should be covered with a protective shield, and an ophthalmologist should be consulted for further evaluation.

Vitreous Hemorrhage/Endophthalmitis

Vitreous hemorrhage (VH) is one cause of decreased visual acuity that can lead to blindness and complete loss of vision. It occurs at a rate of approximately seven cases per 100,000 people [36]. Patients may complain of "black rain" obscuring their vision from hemorrhaging blood spreading diffusely within the viscous vitreous [10]. Some of the causes of VH include posterior vitreous detachment, diabetic retinopathy, retinal micro aneurysms, vascular tumors, and trauma [10]. US has a sensitivity and specificity of 84.6% and 96.5%, respectively, for detecting VH [28]. The sonographic appearance depends on its age and severity: recent and mild VH appear as small dots or linear areas of areas of low reflective opacities that are mobile with ocular movements, whereas more severe and older hemorrhages appear to have dependent echogenic layers within the posterior chamber [21]. Movement of the eye will demonstrate a swirling or tumbling of the echogenic contents within the posterior chamber, otherwise known as a "swirl sign" [21, 22].

Endophthalmitis can appear similar to a VH, with a hyperechoic vitreous opacification with convection movements and movements with ocular motion. Different organisms will have different appearance on US, with streptococcal species tending to produce a denser, more hyperechoic signal, while gram-negative species are associated with minimal vitreous opacities [37]. Endophthalmitis can be difficult to distinguish from VH, and if there is any concern for infection, an emergent ophthalmologic evaluation is recommended.

Elevated Intracranial Pressure/Enlarged Optic Nerve Sheath Diameter

Ocular US has been shown to be an effective method to evaluate the optic nerve sheath diameter (ONSD) which is highly correlated with elevated intracranial pressure (eICP), allowing for measurement of the ONSD to be a rapid and noninvasive means of evaluating patients with traumatic head injuries and patients who are at risk of nontraumatic causes of eICP (e.g., spontaneous intracranial hemorrhage, cerebral vascular accidents, idiopathic intracranial hypertension, meningitis, encephalitis, post-resuscitation syndrome following cardiac arrest, liver failure, large cerebral masses or space occupying lesions, increased cerebrospinal fluid production, obstruction of the ventricular system, cerebral edema, and craniosynostosis) [38, 39] when CT is not readily available. This is of great importance, as undiagnosed eICP can lead to significant morbidity and increased mortality through secondary ischemic insult or brainstem herniation. For each 1 mm increase in ONSD, overall hospital mortality is increased twofold [40]. It should be noted, however, that even though there is high correlation between the ONSD and eICP, it is impossible to draw conclusions as to the actual intracranial pressure from the ONSD, as the relationship between ONSD and cerebrospinal pressure is unknown in the individual cases (elasticity of the optic nerve sheath), a normal variability of the ONSD exists from person to person, and the baseline normal ONSD is usually unknown [41].

The reason an elevated ONSD is correlated with increased intracranial pressure (ICP) is that the space between the optic nerve and the optic nerve sheath is continuous with the cerebral subarachnoid space. Any pathology that increases the volume or pressure of this space will transmit the change in pressure and volume to the space within the optic nerve sheath. The ONSD changes most in the most anterior portion, just behind the globe [42]. This is the same pathophysiology that leads to papilledema; however, the funduscopic exam is frequently difficult and might be impossible in the setting of trauma. US has the potential to reliably and accurately measure the optic nerve sheath [43]. Studies have shown emergency physicians are capable of accurately measuring the ONSD using a bedside US machine [44] and that the measurement of the ONSD can be easily taught to novices [39]. However, the full clinical picture should be evaluated as there are ocular conditions that can mimic papilledema, such as optic nerve tumors and optic nerve head drusen [45].

The measurement of the ONSD should be taken at a depth of 3 mm behind the retina, as this is the area that will show the greatest change [46] due to eICP and also provides a consistent location for measurement across multiple operators and scans [47]. The US probe should be manipulated in such a manner as to have the US waves travel parallel to the optic nerve. Once the optic nerve sheath is identified, the probe should be fanned to find the widest part of the sheath. The measurement should be made perpendicular to the direction of the nerve, and multiple (two to three) measurements should be made and averaged together.

There are 16 studies that have looked at the relationship between ONSD measurements and eICP [42, 48–63]. A summary of these articles can be found in Table 14.1. Despite much effort dedicated toward finding the efficacy of using an ONSD measurement to rule out or rule in eICP, there are no large trials. There is also no consistent ONSD cutoff across the studies with a range 4.7–5.9 mm; however, of those studies conducted in the emergency department, all but one uses a cutoff of 5.0 mm, and the one that is different uses 4.7 mm. Overall sensitivities range from 70% to 100%, and specificities range from 44% to 100%, which is the same range looking only at the studies performed in the emergency department setting. In studies with TBI, the sensitivities range from 86% to 100% and the specificities from 75% to 100%. A more

TABLE 14.1 Summary of studies evaluating the ultrasonic measurement of the optic nerve sheath diameter (ONSD) as a predictor of elevated intracranial pressure (eICP)

Study	Setting/ patient population	Study size	ONSD cutoff	Comparator	Disability	Sensi-tivity (%)	Spec-ificity (%)	Likelihood ratio for a positive test	Likelihood ratio for a negative test	Negative predictive value (%)	Positive predictive value (%)	Area under the curve	ONSD/ comparator correlation coefficient
Blaivas et al. [48]	Emergency department	35	5.0 mm	Computed tomography	Blunt TBI and suspected ICH	100	95	20.0	0	100	93	–	–
Tayal et al. [49]	Emergency department	59	5.0 mm	Computed tomography	Traumatic head injury	100	63	2.7	0	100	30	–	–
Geeraerts et al. [50]	ICU	31	5.9 mm	Invasive ICP monitoring	Severe TBI, SAH, ICH, CVA	87	94	14.5	0.14	88	93	0.94	0.68
Geeraerts et al. [51]	Neuro ICU	37	5.8 mm	Invasive ICP monitoring	Severe TBI, SAH, ICH, CVA	95	79	4.5	0.06	–	–	0.91	0.71
Soldatos et al. [52]	ICU	50	5.7 mm	Noninvasive and invasive ICP monitoring	Brain injury	74.10	100	Undefined	0.26	–	–	0.93	0.68

TABLE 14.1 (continued)

Study	Setting/patient population	Study size	ONSD cutoff	Comparator	Disability	Sensitivity (%)	Specificity (%)	Likelihood ratio for a positive test	Likelihood ratio for a negative test	Negative predictive value (%)	Positive predictive value (%)	Area under the curve	ONSD/comparator correlation coefficient
Kimberly et al. [53]	ED and ICU	15	5.0 mm	Invasive ICP monitoring	Patients with invasive ICP monitoring	88	93	12.6	0.13	–	–	0.93	0.59
Goel et al. [54]	Patients admitted with head trauma	100	5.0 mm	Computed tomography	Traumatic head injury	98.6	92.6	13.3	0.02	96.5	97.3	–	–
Moretti et al. [55]	ICU	53	5.2 mm	Invasive ICP monitoring	ICH, SAH	94	76	3.9	0.08	–	–	0.89	0.69
Moretti et al. [64]	ICU	63	5.2 mm	Invasive ICP monitoring	Spontaneous intracranial hemorrhage	93.1	73.8	3.6	0.09	–	–	0.925	0.7
Major et al. [57]	Emergency department	26	5.0 mm	Computed tomography	TBI, CVA, SAH, SDH, EDH, tumor	86	100	Undefined	0.14	–	–	–	–

Bäuerle et al. [58]	Not specified	10	5.8 mm	Lumbar puncture	Ideopathic intracranial hypertension	90	84	5.6	0.12	–	–	0.92	–
Qayyum et al. [42]	Emergency department	24	5.0 mm	Computed tomography	TBI, clinical signs of eICP	100	75	4	0.00	100	95.40	–	–
Frumin et al. [59]	Neuro ICU	27	5.2 mm	External ventricular device	Invasively monitored patients	83.3	100	Undefined	0.17	95.5	100	0.87	0.4
Caffery et al. [60]	Emergency department	51	5.0 mm	Lumbar puncture	Non-traumatic eICP	75	44	1.3	0.57	–	–	0.69	0.53
Maissan et al. [61]	ICU	18	5.0 mm	Invasive ICP monitoring	Traumatic head injury	94	90	9.4	0.07	–	–	0.99	0.90
Komut et al. [62]	Emergency department	100	4.7 mm	Computed tomography	Non-traumatic intracranial lesions	70	86	5	0.35	–	–	0.86	–

ICU intensive care unit, *TBI* traumatic brain injury, *SAH* subarachnoid hemorrhage, *ICH* intracranial hemorrhage, *CVA* cerebral vascular accident, *SDH* subdural hemorrhage, *EDH* extradural hemorrhage, *eICP* elevated intracranial pressure, *ED* emergency department indolent chronic presentation of IIH or other nontraumatic cause of eICP may be to blame for the decreased sensitivities and specificities observed in the studies which only identified nontraumatic causes of eICP. Interobserver variation ranges from 0.20 to 0.25 mm [56, 64].

Difference in ONSD measurements between eyes can suggest mass effect. A 0.45 mm difference between the ONSD measurements of each eye is highly suggestive of an intracranial lesion with an area under the curve of 0.794 and a sensitivity and specificity of 80% and 60%, respectively, with the side of the larger ONSD corresponding to the side of the intracranial lesion. ONSD is also higher in patients with midline shift [62].

US of the ONSD can also be used in pediatric patients for evaluation of eICP. Normal ranges of ONSD in pediatric patients vary based on ethnicity (2.0–4.35) [65–67]. Only two papers have looked at the sensitivity and specificity of ONSD measurements in children as a means of evaluating for eICP, with cutoffs of 4.2–4.5 mm displaying sensitivities of 93–100% and specificities 86–100% [65]. Newman et al. found that the ONSD increases with age, particularly in the first year of life, and suggested a normal cutoff of 4 mm in patients younger than 1 year of age. The majority of this change happens in the first 5 years of life, with minimal increase from 5 to 16 years. Effectively, the adult size is effectively reached between 4 and 5 years of age [47]. As such, a cutoff of 4.5 mm in patients between 1 year and 4 years of age and 5.0 mm thereafter has been proposed [68, 69], although using a cutoff of 4.5 mm until age 15, when the ONSD should have reached adult size, may yield a higher sensitivity [22].

There is a high degree of correlation between ONSD and ICP, but whether the ONSD can be used as a reliable method to rule out eICP when a CT scanner is not available has not yet been fully determined. Unfortunately, as the ONSD has minimal change with increases of ICP as low was 8–10 mmHg, and even though the sheath can increase by more than 50%, the inherent elasticity of each individual's sheath is not known, and there may always be factors that prohibit a consistently high sensitivity.

Dynamic Ocular Exam

Frequently a facial trauma patient's eyelids will be significantly edematous, precluding a thorough ocular examination for even the most basic of elements: extraocular muscles (EOM) and pupillary light reflex (PLR). Prior to US, if the periorbital skin and eyelid were so edematous that the ocular exam could not be performed, then the eyelids were pried apart with retractors so that a visual inspection could be made. This carries the risk of globe perforation and corneal abrasion, and it frequently causes pain. More recently US has been proposed as a nontraumatic means of assessing the EOM and PLR [70].

To evaluate EOM, the patient is positioned as they would be for any ocular US evaluation. Once a mid-globe view is attained, the patient is instructed to move their eyes in all four directions, which can be visualized in real time. Additionally, the probe can be held parallel to any of the primary EOM movements to maintain constant visualization of the lens and pupil throughout the range of motion. The pupillary light reflex exam should be performed in a dark room. The transducer is placed on the superior portion of the patient's closed eye in the transverse plane and angled inferiorly. The probe is fanned to find an image that contains the entire iris with the anechoic pupil in the center. A light is shined in the opposite eye, and if normal, the pupil of the affected eye should be visualized constricting. Measurements of the pupil size before and after light stimulation can be made. In a situation where both eyes are affected, a bright light can be shown through the closed eyelid, and both eyes can be examined [71].

Pearls/Pitfalls

- Use copious amounts to ultrasound gel to prevent pressure increasing the intraocular pressure and to help capture the best images with the least amount of artifacts.

- If there is any concern for or signs of globe rupture, do not ultrasound the eye.
- Numerous artifacts (e.g., ring down, reverberation, air scattering, shadowing) may interfere with the examination and may be mistaken for pathology.
- Use the least amount of energy for the shortest amount of time to prevent undue harm from the study, especially when using color Doppler imaging or pulse-wave Doppler which increase the energy used.
- If it is unclear whether an object is artifact or pathology, adjusting the gain and transducer angle can help differentiate the two. If still in doubt, increasing the amount of gel may help reduce the amount of artifact.

References

1. Sharma R, Brunette DD. Rosen's emergency medicine concepts and clinical practice. 8th ed. Philadelphia, PA: Saunders; 2014. p. 909. Chapter 71.
2. Romaniuk VM. Ocular trauma and other catastrophes. Emerg Med Clin North Am. 2013;31(2):399–411.
3. Colby K. Management of open globe injuries. Int Ophthalmol Clin. 1999;39(1):59–69.
4. Rocha KM, Martins EN, Melo LA Jr, et al. Outpatient management of traumatic hyphema in children: prospective evaluation. J AAPOS. 2004;8(4):357–61.
5. Wu EH, et al. Self-confidence in and perceived utility of the physical examination: a comparison of medical students, residents, and faculty internists. J Gen Intern Med. 2007;22(12):1725–30.
6. Ritchie JV, Horne ST, Perry J, Gay D. Ultrasound triage of ocular blast injury in the military emergency department. Mil Med. 2012;177(2):174–8.
7. Gay DAT, et al. Ultrasound of penetrating ocular injury in a combat environment. Clin Radiol. 2013;68(1):82–4.
8. Russell TC, Crawford PF. Ultrasound in the austere environment: a review of the history, indications, and specifications. Mil Med. 2013;178(1):21–8.
9. American College of Emergency Physicians. Policy Statement on Ultrasound Guidelines: Emergency, Point-of-Care, and Clinical Ultrasound Guidelines in Medicine, June 2016. https://www.acep.

org/Clinical---Practice-Management/Ultrasound-Guidelines--Emergency,-Point-of-care,-and-Clinical-Ultrasound-Guidelines-in-Medicine/?__taxonomyid=471332. Accessed 5 Nov 2018.

10. Bedi DG, Gombos DS, Ng CS, Singh S. Sonography of the eye. AJR Am J Roentgenol. 2006;187(4):1061–72.

11. Blaivas M, Theodoro D, Sierzenski PR. A study of bedside ocular ultrasonography in the emergency department. Acad Emerg Med. 2002;9(8):791–9.

12. Bioeffects Committee of the American Institute of Ultrasound in Medicine. American Institute of Ultrasound in Medicine consensus report on potential bioeffects of diagnostic ultrasound executive summary. J Ultrasound Med. 2008;27(4):503–15.

13. Duck FA. Hazards, risks and safety of diagnostic ultrasound. Med Eng Phys. 2008;30(10):1338–48.

14. Hershkovitz R, Sheiner E, Mazor M. Ultrasound in obstetrics: a review of safety. Eur J Obstet Gynecol Reprod Biol. 2002;101(1):15–8.

15. Barnett SB, Ter Haar GR, Ziskin MC, Rott HD, Duck FA, Maeda K. International recommendation and guidelines for the safe use of diagnostic ultrasound in medicine. Ultrasound Med Biol. 2000;26:355–66.

16. Palte HD, Gayer S, Arrieta E, et al. Are ultrasound-guided ophthalmic blocks injurious to the eye? A comparative rabbit model study of two ultrasound devices evaluating intraorbital thermal and structural changes. Anesth Analg. 2012;115(1):194–201.

17. Silverman RH, Lizzi FL, Ursea BG, et al. Safety levels for exposure of cornea and lens to very high-frequency ultrasound. J Ultrasound Med. 2001;20(9):979–86.

18. Nelson TR, Fowlkes JB, Abramowicz JS, Church CC. Ultrasound biosafety considerations for the practicing sonographer and sonologist. J Ultrasound Med. 2009;28(2):139–50.

19. Park DJ, Karesh JW. Topographic anatomy of the eye: an overview. In: Duane's foundations of clinical ophthalmology. Philadelphia, PA: Lippincott Williams & Wilkins; 2006.

20. Roth KR, Gafni-Pappas G. Unique method of ocular ultrasound using transparent dressings. J Emerg Med. 2011;40(6):658–60.

21. Adhikari SR. Sonoguide website at: http://www.sonoguide.com/smparts_ocular.html. Accessed 4 Aug 2016.

22. Kilker BA, Holst JM, Hoffmann B. Bedside ocular ultrasound in the emergency department. Eur J Emerg Med. 2014;21(4):246–53.

23. D'Amico DJ. Clinical practice. Primary retinal detachment. N Engl J Med. 2008;359(22):2346–54.

24. Teismann N, Shah S, Nagdev A. Focus on: ultrasound for acute retinal detachment. Irving, TX: ACEP News; 2009.
25. Yoonessi R, Hussain A, Jang TB. Bedside ocular ultrasound for the detection of retinal detachment in the emergency department. Acad Emerg Med. 2010;17(9):913–7.
26. Shinar Z, Chan L, Orlinsky M. Use of ocular ultrasound for the evaluation of retinal detachment. J Emerg Med. 2011;40(1):53–7.
27. Jacobsen B, Lahham S, Lahham S, Patel A, Spann S, Fox JC. Retrospective review of ocular point-of-care ultrasound for detection of retinal detachment. West J Emerg Med. 2016;17(2):196–200.
28. Imran S, Amin S, Daula MI. Imaging in ocular trauma optimizing the use of ultrasound and computerised tomography. Pak J Ophthalmol. 2011;27(3):146–51.
29. Ido M, Osawa S, Fukukita M, et al. The use of colour Doppler imaging in the diagnosis of retinal detachment. Eye (Lond). 2007;21(11):1375–8.
30. Jarrett WH. Dislocation of the lens. A study of 166 hospitalized cases. Arch Ophthalmol. 1967;78:289–96.
31. Nelson LB, Maumenee IH. Ectopia lentis. Surv Ophthalmol. 1982;27(3):143–60.
32. Frasure SE, Saul T, Lewiss RE. Bedside ultrasound diagnosis of vitreous hemorrhage and traumatic lens dislocation. Am J Emerg Med. 2013;31(6):1002.e1–2.
33. Ojaghi Haghighi SH, Morteza Begi HR, Sorkhabi R, et al. Diagnostic accuracy of ultrasound in detection of traumatic lens dislocation. Emerg (Tehran). 2014;2(3):121–4.
34. Eken C, Yuruktumen A, Yildiz G. Ultrasound diagnosis of traumatic lens dislocation. J Emerg Med. 2013;44(1):e109–10.
35. Leo M, Carmody K. Sonography assessment of acute ocular pathology. Ultrasound Clin. 2011;6(2):227–34.
36. Rabinowitz R, Yagev R, Shoham A, Lifshitz T. Comparison between clinical and ultrasound findings in patients with vitreous hemorrhage. Eye (Lond). 2004;18(3):253–6.
37. Kohanim S, Daniels AB, Huynh N, Eliott D, Chodosh J. Utility of ultrasonography in diagnosing infectious endophthalmitis in patients with media opacities. Semin Ophthalmol. 2012;27:242–5.
38. Girisgin AS, Kalkan E, Kocak S, Cander B, Gul M, Semiz M. The role of optic nerve ultrasonography in the diagnosis of elevated intracranial pressure. Emerg Med J. 2007;24(4):251–4.

39. Potgieter DW, Kippin A, Ngu F, McKean C. Can accurate ultra-sonographic measurement of the optic nerve sheath diameter (a non-invasive measure of intracranial pressure) be taught to novice operators in a single training session? Anaesth Intensive Care. 2011;39(1):95–100.

40. Sekhon MS, McBeth P, Zou J, et al. Association between optic nerve sheath diameter and mortality in patients with severe traumatic brain injury. Neurocrit Care. 2014;21(2):245–52.

41. Hansen HC, Helmke K. Validation of the optic nerve sheath response to changing cerebrospinal fluid pressure: ultra-sound findings during intrathecal infusion tests. J Neurosurg. 1997;87(1):34–40.

42. Qayyum H, Ramlakhan S. Can ocular ultrasound predict intra-cranial hypertension? A pilot diagnostic accuracy evaluation in a UK emergency department. Eur J Emerg Med. 2013;20(2):91–7.

43. Stone MB. Ultrasound diagnosis of papilledema and increased intracranial pressure in pseudotumor cerebri. Am J Emerg Med. 2009;27(3):376.e1–2.

44. Hassen GW, Bruck I, Donahue J, et al. Accuracy of optic nerve sheath diameter measurement by emergency physicians using bedside ultrasound. J Emerg Med. 2015;48(4):450–7.

45. Rifenburg RP, Williams JJ. Optic nerve head drusen: a case of false-positive papilledema discovered by ocular ultrasound in the emergency department. Crit Ultrasound J. 2010;2(2):75–6.

46. Helmke K, Hansen HC. Fundamentals of transorbital sono-graphic evaluation of optic nerve sheath expansion under intracranial hypertension II. Patient study. Pediatr Radiol. 1996;26(10):706–10.

47. Newman WD, Hollman AS, Dutton GN, Carachi R. Measurement of optic nerve sheath diameter by ultrasound: a means of detect-ing acute raised intracranial pressure in hydrocephalus. Br J Ophthalmol. 2002;86(10):1109–13.

48. Blaivas M, Theodoro D, Sierzenski PR. Elevated intracranial pressure detected by bedside emergency ultrasonography of the optic nerve sheath. Acad Emerg Med. 2003;10(4):376–81.

49. Tayal VS, Neulander M, Norton HJ, Foster T, Saunders T, Blaivas M. Emergency department sonographic measurement of optic nerve sheath diameter to detect findings of increased intracra-nial pressure in adult head injury patients. Ann Emerg Med. 2007;49(4):508–14.

50. Geeraerts T, Launey Y, Martin L, et al. Ultrasonography of the optic nerve sheath may be useful for detecting raised intracranial pressure after severe brain injury. Intensive Care Med. 2007;33(10):1704–11.
51. Geeraerts T, Merceron S, Benhamou D, Vigué B, Duranteau J. Noninvasive assessment of intracranial pressure using ocular sonography in neurocritical care patients. Crit Care. 2008;12(2):1.
52. Soldatos T, Karakitsos D, Chatzimichail K, Papathanasiou M, Gouliamos A, Karabinis A. Optic nerve sonography in the diagnostic evaluation of adult brain injury. Crit Care. 2008;12(3):R67.
53. Kimberly HH, Shah S, Marill K, Noble V. Correlation of optic nerve sheath diameter with direct measurement of intracranial pressure. Acad Emerg Med. 2008;15(2):201–4.
54. Goel RS, Goyal NK, Dharap SB, Kumar M, Gore MA. Utility of optic nerve ultrasonography in head injury. Injury. 2008;39(5):519–24.
55. Moretti R, Pizzi B. Optic nerve ultrasound for detection of intracranial hypertension in intracranial hemorrhage patients. J Neurosurg Anesthesiol. 2009;21(1):16–20.
56. Ballantyne SA, O'Neill G, Hamilton R, Hollman AS. Observer variation in the sonographic measurement of optic nerve sheath diameter in normal adults. Eur J Ultrasound. 2002;15(3):145–9.
57. Major R, Girling S, Boyle A. Ultrasound measurement of optic nerve sheath diameter in patients with a clinical suspicion of raised intracranial pressure. Emerg Med J. 2011;28(8):679–81.
58. Bäuerle J, Nedelmann M. Sonographic assessment of the optic nerve sheath in idiopathic intracranial hypertension. J Neurol. 2011;258(11):2014–9.
59. Frumin E, Schlang J, Wiechmann W, et al. Prospective analysis of single operator sonographic optic nerve sheath diameter measurement for diagnosis of elevated intracranial pressure. West J Emerg Med. 2014;15(2):217–20.
60. Caffery TS, Perret JN, Musso MW, Jones GN. Optic nerve sheath diameter and lumbar puncture opening pressure in nontrauma patients suspected of elevated intracranial pressure. Am J Emerg Med. 2014;32(12):1513–5.
61. Maissan IM, Dirven PJAC, Haitsma IK, Hoeks SE, Gommers D, Stolker RJ. Ultrasonographic measured optic nerve sheath diameter as an accurate and quick monitor for changes in intracranial pressure. J Neurosurg. 2015;123(3):743–7.
62. Komut E, Kozacı N, Sönmez BM, Yılmaz F, Komut S, Yıldırım ZN, Beydilli İ, Yel C. Bedside sonographic measurement of optic

nerve sheath diameter as a predictor of intracranial pressure in ED. Am J Emerg Med. 2016;34(6):963–7.

63. Kazdal H, Kanat A, Findik H, et al. Transorbital ultrasonographic measurement of optic nerve sheath diameter for intracranial midline shift in patients with head trauma. World Neurosurg. 2016;85:292–7.

64. Moretti R, Pizzi B, Cassini F, Vivaldi N. Reliability of optic nerve ultrasound for the evaluation of patients with spontaneous intracranial hemorrhage. Neurocrit Care. 2009;11(3):406–10.

65. Beare NAV, Kampondeni S, Glover SJ, et al. Detection of raised intracranial pressure by ultrasound measurement of optic nerve sheath diameter in African children. Tropical Med Int Health. 2008;13(11):1400–4.

66. Malayeri AA, Bavarian S, Mehdizadeh M. Sonographic evaluation of optic nerve diameter in children with raised intracranial pressure. J Ultrasound Med. 2005;24(2):143–7.

67. Ballantyne J, Hollman AS, Hamilton R, Bradnam MS, Carachi R, Young DG, Dutton GN. Transorbital optic nerve sheath ultrasonography in normal children. Clin Radiol. 1999;54(11):740–2.

68. Le A, Hoehn ME, Smith ME, Spentzas T, Schlappy D, Pershad J. Bedside sonographic measurement of optic nerve sheath diameter as a predictor of increased intracranial pressure in children. Ann Emerg Med. 2009;53(6):785–91.

69. Moretti R, Pizzi B. Ultrasonography of the optic nerve in neurocritically ill patients. Acta Anaesthesiol Scand. 2011;55(6):644–52.

70. Chiao L, Sharipov S, Sargsyan AE, Melton S, Hamilton DR, McFarlin K, Dulchavsky SA. Ocular examination for trauma; clinical ultrasound aboard the International Space Station. J Trauma Acute Care Surg. 2005;58(5):885–9.

71. Harries A, Shah S, Teismann N, Price D, Nagdev A. Ultrasound assessment of extraocular movements and pupillary light reflex in ocular trauma. Am J Emerg Med. 2010;28(8):956–9.

Chapter 15
Ocular Imaging

Paul Basel

Obtaining proper imaging for patients with ocular complaints is crucial to an emergency physician's management of ocular disorders. Ultrasound imaging has been previously discussed. Ultrasound provides the benefit of rapid bedside diagnostics; however, it is only useful in a handful of diagnosis and does not provide the sensitivity and detailed imaging required for many diagnosis and operative planning. Other tools at an emergency physician's disposal include plain radiography, CT scanning and MRI (although this may be difficult at some facilities). Imaging options will be discussed based on clinical scenarios.

Trauma

CT orbits without contrast are the gold standard for ocular imaging in trauma [1]. When evaluating a patient with ocular trauma, a number of questions need to be considered by the emergency physician in order to properly inform imaging choices.

P. Basel, MD
Department of Emergency Medicine, San Antonio Uniformed
Services Health Education Consortium, San Antonio, TX, USA

© Springer International Publishing AG, part of Springer   273
Nature 2018
B. Long, A. Koyfman (eds.), *Handbook of Emergency
Ophthalmology*, https://doi.org/10.1007/978-3-319-78945-3_15

Is There Concern for an Open Globe?

Open globe or suspicion of an open globe is a contraindication to ocular ultrasound [1, 2] and will likely require more advanced imaging. Open globe should be suspected based on history and physical examination. Examination findings concerning for open globe include a peaked pupil, obvious herniated ocular contents, and a positive Seidel's sign. Unfortunately, physical examination is poorly sensitive and is often difficult due to significant periorbital swelling and patient cooperation. Patients with significant ocular trauma in whom physical examination is inadequate to evaluate for open globe should have advanced imaging to evaluate for open globe and associated injuries. CT orbits are the preferred imaging modality for evaluating open globe given the speed and safety of the test [2]. Unfortunately, the test has relatively poor sensitivity for ruptured globe. Reported sensitivities and specificities range from 56% to 76% and 79% to 100%, respectively [3–5]. Therefore the emergency clinician should remain suspicious of an open globe injury despite negative imaging if history or physical examination suggests the diagnosis.

Is There Concern for Penetrating Foreign Body?

If intraocular foreign body (IOFB) is suspected based on history or physical, MRI should be avoided until metallic foreign body can be ruled out [1]. Initial imaging studies for suspected IOFB include X-ray and CT scan. Prior to the advent of CT scanning, X-ray was the primary imaging modality for detecting radiopaque IOFBs. Unfortunately, X-ray lacks sensitivity, especially for nonmetallic objects [1]. Several studies have evaluated plain radiography in the setting of IOFB and found sensitivity for metallic objects between 69 and 90%, for glass 71 and 77%, and a dismal 0 and 15% for objects such as wood and graphite [6]. In contrast, studies evaluating CT scanning for metallic foreign bodies have found excellent sensitivity and specificity reported at 100% for both [7]. Unfortunately, nonmetallic objects remain more difficult to identify. In a study comparing CT, MRI, and US for identifying glass IOFBs in porcine eyes, CT was found to be the most sensitive with 96% detection rate for glass objects over 1.5 mm but only 48% detection rate for glass 0.5 mm or less in size [8]. Wooden IOFB is difficult to diagnose using any imaging modality, and evidence for detection of these rare foreign objects is restricted to case reports and series. Wood can appear similar to air or fat on CT; therefore, it is imperative to alert your radiologist if there is concern for a wooden IOFB [1]. If CT is equivocal or negative and suspicion for wooden IOFB persists, MRI or US may demonstrate an object missed by CT [9].

In the absence of a history or physical examination concerning for IOFB, it may be reasonable to eliminate imaging to rule out IOFB. In a retrospective review of patients who underwent orbital X-ray to rule out IOFB at a single institution, patients were stratified by suspicion for IOFB based on physical examination. Eight hundred and eighty patients were identified in which there was no concern on physical examination for penetrating ocular trauma; radiographs in this population found zero IOFBs [6]. In a second retrospective study in patients with no evidence of penetrating trauma, 177 had plain radiographs performed and 9 had CT orbit performed. In this group, one IOFB was identified on X-ray which was later found to be a false positive; zero IOFBs were found on CT orbits [7]. These studies indicate it may be reasonable to forgo imaging in patients with no evidence of penetrating trauma. However, the emergency clinician should maintain a high degree of suspicion when history indicates high-risk activities (EG hammering, metal grinding, etc.) or when physical examination is limited due to periorbital swelling or patient cooperation.

Is There an Orbital Wall Fracture?

Damage to the bony orbit is common in orbital trauma. Plain radiographs can be used to successfully diagnose many orbital fractures; however, sensitivity is low between 50 and

78% [1, 10]. CT orbits provide excellent resolution of the bony architecture of the orbit as well as soft tissue to evaluate for other injuries or muscle entrapment. Radiographs are rarely used given the speed and accuracy of CT.

Bottom Line

CT orbit is the preferred imaging modality in trauma. CT is insensitive for diagnosing open globe. If the history or physical examination suggests open globe but imaging is negative, the patient may still need surgical exploration due to the poor sensitivity of the test.

In cases of suspected IOFB, CT scanning of orbits is the preferred and most sensitive modality. MRI should not be performed unless metallic IOFB has been ruled out. If suspicion for IOFB remains high despite negative CT scanning, MRI or US may be reasonable to evaluate for less common objects such as wood. If there is no suspicion for IOFB based on history and physical examination, it may be reasonable to forgo imaging to rule out IOFB.

Medical

The majority of medical emergencies of the eye are clinical diagnosis made with a thorough history and physical examination including slit lamp and tonometry. However, there are several emergent medical conditions that warrant advanced imaging. MRI with contrast provides the greatest soft tissue detail of the eye and is often the best choice for imaging of medical conditions of the eye [11]. Time and equipment constraints often make MRI impractical in the emergency department. CT orbits with contrast provide greater speed and availability and may be an adequate test for many medical diagnoses. Plain radiography does not have a significant role in evaluation of medical disease of the eye. Ocular ultrasound has been discussed in the previous chapter and is extremely useful for several ocular medical conditions such

as retinal detachment, vitreous hemorrhage, and lens dislocation. These will not be reviewed here.

Preseptal Cellulitis and Orbital Cellulitis

Orbital cellulitis is an ocular emergency that often requires
surgical intervention; however, clinically distinguishing it
from preseptal cellulitis can be difficult [12]. Advanced imaging can help the clinician evaluate for orbital involvement.
Preseptal and orbital cellulitis are primarily diseases of children, and therefore ionizing radiation should be avoided
whenever practical. CT and MRI are the primary modalities
available to evaluate for these conditions [12]. Historically,
plain films of sinuses were used to evaluate for sinus opacification, given that the majority of orbital cellulitis occurs due
to extension from sinus disease. This is no longer performed,
as no correlation between sinus opacification and infection
has been shown [13]. CT orbits with IV contrast (include
head if concerned for intracranial extension) are often the
study of choice in the acute setting given the study's speed,
availability, and cost [14]. However, MRI head and orbits with
and without contrast provide the greatest soft tissue detail
and may be preferable, especially in the pediatric setting [11,
15]. MRI may not be available at all institutions and may
require sedation for pediatric studies.

The decision to obtain advanced imaging based on physical examination can be difficult, and little data exists to guide
physicians. A recent retrospective review of 918 patients with
suspected orbital cellulitis attempted to define high-risk features that would require imaging. In this study, proptosis, pain
with extraocular movements, edema extending beyond the
eyelid, and ANC >10,000 were high-risk features necessitating imaging [16]. Unfortunately, lack of these symptoms did
not rule out orbital involvement. Additionally, patients with
suspected orbital cellulitis may be successfully treated with
antibiotics alone, thereby eliminating the need for imaging.
This was illustrated in a case series of nine patients with

CT-proven orbital subperiosteal abscesses [17]. In this study surgical intervention was withheld unless patients had progressive optic nerve involvement 24–36 h after starting antibiotics. Only one patient required surgical intervention. This small study indicates it may be reasonable to admit and observe patients suspected to have orbital cellulitis on IV antibiotics and reserve imaging for those who do not respond to medical therapy. Further study is required to validate this treatment plan.

Optic Neuritis

Optic neuritis is a common condition that is characterized by painful monocular vision loss. While optic neuritis is typically a clinical diagnosis, advanced imaging can help support the diagnosis or suggest other causes [18]. Imaging is also indicated with atypical presentations of optic neuritis (such as bilateral symptoms, painless presentation) as intracranial pathology can present similarly [19]. If imaging is pursued, MRI brain and orbits with gadolinium contrast is the study of choice [18, 20–22]. Including brain in the image can evaluate for rarer intracranial causes of symptoms. In a retrospective case series review of 107 patients diagnosed with optic neuritis, MRI demonstrated a sensitivity of 94.4% [20]. While optic neuritis remains a clinical diagnosis, patients with atypical symptoms and no evidence of optic neuritis on MRI warrant further workup, likely by an ophthalmologist for causes of vision loss.

Bottom Line

The majority of medical conditions do not require advanced imaging. When advanced imaging is required, MRI with contrast provides the greatest soft tissue detail; however, CT orbits with contrast are often an acceptable choice. Ocular ultrasound is an extremely useful tool for the diagnosis of several medical conditions such as retinal detachment, vitreous hemorrhage, and lens dislocation (please see previous chapter).

When evaluating for post-septal cellulitis, MRI orbits with contrast and CT orbits with contrast are both adequate imaging choices. Consider MRI in the pediatric population to limit radiation exposure. Physical exam can rule out post-septal cellulitis in many cases; when the diagnosis is unclear, imaging is indicated.

The diagnosis of optic neuritis can be made clinically. Atypical presentations may warrant imaging for other possible causes. MRI brain and orbits with contrast can confirm the diagnosis or demonstrate alternative diagnosis.

References

1. Kubal WS. Imaging of orbital trauma. Radiographics. 2008;28(6):1729–39. https://doi.org/10.1148/rg.286085523.
2. Sung EK, Nadgir RN, Fujita A, et al. Injuries of the globe: what can the radiologist offer? Radiographics. 2014;34(3):764–76. https://doi.org/10.1148/rg.343135120.
3. Yuan WH, Hsu HC, Cheng HC, et al. CT of globe rupture: analysis and frequency of findings. Am J Roentgenol. 2014;202(5):1100–7. https://doi.org/10.2214/AJR.13.11010.
4. Joseph DP, Pieramici DJ, Beauchamp NJ. Computed tomography in the diagnosis and prognosis of open-globe injuries. Ophthalmology. 2000;107:1899–906.
5. Arey ML, Mootha VV, Whittemore AR, Chason DP, Blomquist PH. Computed tomography in the diagnosis of occult open-globe injuries. Ophthalmology. 2007;114(8):1448–52. https://doi.org/10.1016/j.ophtha.2006.10.051.
6. Bray LC, Griffiths PG. The value of plain radiography in suspected intraocular foreign body. Eye. 1991;5:751–4.
7. Saeed a CL, Malone DE, Beatty S. Plain X-ray and computed tomography of the orbit in cases and suspected cases of intraocular foreign body. Eye (Lond). 2008;22(11):1373–7. https://doi.org/10.1038/sj.eye.6702876.
8. Gor DM, Kirsch CF, Leen J, Turbin R, Von Hagen S, et al. Am J Roentgenol.2001;177(5):1199–203.doi:0361–803X/01/1775–1199.

9. Nagae LM, Katowitz WR, Bilaniuk LT, Anninger WV, Pollock AN. Radiological detection of intraorbital wooden foreign bodies. Pediatr Emerg Care. 2011;27(9):895–6. https://doi.org/10.1097/PEC.0b013e31822d3df2.

10. Brady SM, McMann MA, Mazzoli RA, Bushley DM, Ainbinder DJ, Carroll RB. The diagnosis and management of orbital blow-out fractures: update 2001. Am J Emerg Med. 2001;19(2):147–54. https://doi.org/10.1053/ajem.2001.21315.

11. Wippold II FJ, Cornelius RS, Berger KL, Broderick DF, Davis PC, Douglas AC, Germano IM, Hadley JA, McDermott MW, Mechtler LL, Smirniotopoulos JG, Waxman AD. ACR appropriateness criteria® orbits, vision and visual loss. 2012.

12. Tintinalli JE, Stapczynski JS, Ma OJ, Yealy DM, Meckler GD, Cline DM. Tintinalli's emergency medicine a comprehensive study guide. New York: McGraw-Hill Education; 2016. p. 2128.

13. Howe L, Jones NS. Guidelines for the management of periorbital cellulitis/abscess. Clin Otolaryngol Allied Sci. 2004;29(6):725–8. https://doi.org/10.1111/j.1365-2273.2004.00889.x.

14. C a LB, Sakai O. Nontraumatic orbital conditions: diagnosis with CT and MR imaging in the emergent setting. Radiographics. 2008;28(6):1741–53. https://doi.org/10.1148/rg.286085515.

15. Lee S, Yen MT. Management of preseptal and orbital cellulitis. Saudi J Ophthalmol. 2011;25(1):21–9. https://doi.org/10.1016/j.sjopt.2010.10.004.

16. Rudloe TF, Harper MB, Prabhu SP, Rahbar R, VanderVeen D, Kimia AA. Acute periorbital infections: who needs emergent imaging? Pediatrics. 2010;125(4):e719–26. https://doi.org/10.1542/peds.2009-1709.

17. Starkey CR, Steele RW. Medical management of orbital cellulitis. Pediatr Infect Dis J. 2001;20(10):1002–5. http://www.ncbi.nlm.nih.gov/pubmed/11642617.

18. Osborne BJ, Volpe NJ. Optic neuritis and risk of MS: differential diagnosis and management. Cleve Clin J Med. 2009;76(3):181–90. https://doi.org/10.3949/ccjm.76a.07268.

19. Lee AG, Lin DJ, Kaufman M, Golnik KC, Vaphiades MS, Eggenberger E. Atypical features prompting neuroimaging in acute optic neuropathy in adults. Can J Ophthalmol. 2000;35(6):325–30. http://www.ncbi.nlm.nih.gov/pubmed/11091914. Accessed 17 Sept 2016.

20. Kupersmith MJ, Alban T, Zeiffer B, Lefton D. Contrast-enhanced MRI in acute optic neuritis: relationship to visual performance. Brain. 2002;125(Pt 4):812–22. https://doi.org/10.1093/brain/awf087.
21. Rocca MA, Hickman SJ, Bö L, et al. Imaging the optic nerve in multiple sclerosis. Mult Scler. 2005;11(5):537–41. https://doi.org/10.1191/1352458505ms1213oa.
22. Wilhelm H, Schabet M. Diagnostik und Therapie der Optikusneuritis. Dtsch Arztebl. 2015;112:616–26. https://doi.org/10.3238/arztebl.2015.0616.

Chapter 16
Ophthalmology Referral

Ian Bodford

Despite being experts in diagnosing ocular conditions, it can be difficult for an emergency physician to decide when an emergent ophthalmology consultation is required. This is an issue at many hospitals where an ophthalmologist is not available 24 h per day, and the patient would require transfer to a tertiary center for definitive care.

Trauma is generally the primary eye condition requiring emergent consultation. It should be kept in mind that ophthalmology consultation should be deferred until all life-threatening conditions are treated. Concern for penetrating injury of the orbit warrants an emergent consultation, as does a laceration of the eyelid involving the nasolacrimal system, canaliculus, eyelid margin, or tarsal plate [1, 2]. Orbital fractures alone do not require a consultation unless there is loss of vision or a penetrating globe injury; however, a consultation is necessary if an associated retrobulbar hematoma occurs [2]. Immediate consultation is not always needed for chemical burns as long as the pH of the eye can be returned to normal by the emergency physician.

Although a difficult diagnosis to make in the emergency department, if there is any concern for endophthalmitis, a

I. Bodford, MD
St. Francis Hospital, Memphis, TN, USA

© Springer International Publishing AG, part of Springer Nature 2018
B. Long, A. Koyfman (eds.), *Handbook of Emergency Ophthalmology*, https://doi.org/10.1007/978-3-319-78945-3_16

consultation to ophthalmology should be placed, as treatment requires admission for diagnostic evaluation and possible surgery [2]. Acute angle closure glaucoma, especially new diagnoses, requires admission for monitoring of response to medications and intraocular pressures; thus, an emergent consultation is warranted [2]. This should not delay treating the patient with medications by the emergency physician. Uveitis has a broad etiology, including infection, rheumatologic, or malignancy. If deemed severe by the emergency physician, a consultation to ophthalmology, as well as to infectious disease, rheumatology, and oncology, can help make the etiologic diagnosis [2]. Corneal ulceration can lead to corneal perforation with extension of the infection into the anterior chamber. Consultation to an ophthalmologist can help elicit the cause of the ulceration and decrease the chance for permanent vision loss [2]. Orbital cellulitis warrants admission to the hospital for intravenous antibiotics and consultation to an ophthalmologist for vision assessment and treatment management.

Acute vision loss is a worrisome diagnosis in the emergency department. Temporal arteritis can lead to permanent vision loss from retinal ischemia. The gold standard is a temporal artery biopsy for diagnosis, and thus an ophthalmologist is needed for this [2]. Optic neuritis, especially as a first time case, necessitates consultation with an ophthalmologist to rule out other causes of acute vision loss. Irreversible vision loss with central retinal artery occlusion may occur within 4 h of the embolic event. If seen prior to 4 h, assessment by an ophthalmologist should occur, as treatment can be vision saving [2]. Early retinal detachment also needs emergent evaluation by an ophthalmologist for surgical planning.

Not all eye complaints that walk in to the emergency department require an emergent consult to an ophthalmologist. Urgent (within 24 h) or semi-urgent (within 1 week) follow-up at an ophthalmologist or optometrist's office is reasonable in many cases. Generally, emergency physicians are well trained in treating common eye complaints, but it is appropriate for a patient to have close follow-up if the condition could lead to vision loss if mismanaged. Common examples of patients needing urgent follow-up include corneal abrasions and ulcers, herpes keratitis, and bacterial conjunctivitis [1]. If any foreign body is removed from the cornea, urgent follow-up is needed to assess for healing. It is also appropriate to have patients with periorbital cellulitis urgently follow-up with an ophthalmologist to assess for improvement of the infection [1] (Tables 16.1, 16.2, and 16.3).

TABLE 16.1 Conditions requiring emergent consultation	Penetrating globe injury
	Orbital fracture with change in vision/entrapment
	Complex laceration
	Ophthalmologic burn/ exposure
	Endophthalmitis
	Acute angle closure glaucoma
	Corneal ulceration/abrasion affecting visual field
	Orbital cellulitis
	Temporal arteritis
	Retinal detachment
	Acute central retinal artery/ vein occlusion

TABLE 16.2 Conditions requiring referral within 24 h

Abrasion/ulcer not affecting visual field
Orbital fracture without loss of vision/entrapment posterior vitreous detachment
Herpes keratitis
Optic neuritis
Uveitis

TABLE 16.3 Conditions requiring ophthalmologic evaluation within 1 week

Conjunctivitis
Dacryocystitis
Dacryoadenitis
Periorbital cellulitis

References

1. Graves D. Triaging ocular emergencies. BSM Consulting. 2012. http://www.bsmcpss.com/resources/study-guides/OPH%20 03%2014-117.pdf.
2. Magauran B. Conditions requiring emergency ophthalmologic consultation. Emerg Med Clin North Am. 2008;26(1):233–8.

Index

© Springer International Publishing AG, part of Springer
Nature 2018
B. Long, A. Koyfman (eds.), *Handbook of Emergency
Ophthalmology*, https://doi.org/10.1007/978-3-319-78945-3